Vulnerable Populations

Editor

ANGELA RICHARD-EAGLIN

NURSING CLINICS
OF NORTH AMERICA

www.nursing.theclinics.com

Consulting Editor
BENJAMIN SMALLHEER

September 2022 • Volume 57 • Number 3

ELSEVIER

1600 John F. Kennedy Boulevard • Suite 1800 • Philadelphia, Pennsylvania, 19103-2899

http://www.theclinics.com

NURSING CLINICS OF NORTH AMERICA Volume 57, Number 3
September 2022 ISSN 0029-6465, ISBN-13: 978-0-323-98769-1

Editor: Kerry Holland
Developmental Editor: Axell Ivan Jade M. Purificacion

Nursing Clinics of North America (ISSN 0029-6465) is published quarterly by Elsevier Inc., 360 Park Avenue South, New York, NY 10010-1710. Months of issue are March, June, September, and December. Periodicals postage paid at New York, NY and additional mailing offices. Subscription price per year is, $163.00 (US individuals), $689.00 (US institutions), $275.00 (international individuals), $710.00 (international institutions), $231.00 (Canadian individuals), $710.00 (Canadian institutions), $100.00 (US and Canadian students), and $135.00 (international students). To receive student/resident rate, orders must be accompanied by name of affiliated institution, date of term, and the signature of program/residency coordinator on institution letterhead. Orders will be billed at individual rate until proof of status is received. Foreign air speed delivery is included in all *Clinics* subscription prices. All prices are subject to change without notice. **POSTMASTER:** Send address changes to *Nursing Clinics*, Elsevier Health Sciences Division, Subscription Customer Service, 3251 Riverport Lane, Maryland Heights, MO 63043. **Customer Service: Telephone: 1-800-654-2452** (U.S. and Canada); **1-314-447-8871 (outside U.S. and Canada). Fax: 1-314-447-8029. E-mail: journalscustomerservice-usa@elsevier.com** (for print support) and **journalsonlinesupport-usa@elsevier.com** (for online support).

Nursing Clinics of North America is covered in *EMBASE/Excerpta Medica, MEDLINE/PubMed (Index Medicus), Social Sciences Citation Index, Current Contents, ASCA, Cumulative Index to Nursing, RNdex Top 100,* and Allied Health Literature and International Nursing Index (INI).

Contributors

CONSULTING EDITOR

BENJAMIN SMALLHEER, PhD, RN, ACNP-BC, FNP-BC, CCRN, CNE
Associate Clinical Professor, School of Nursing, Duke University, Durham, North Carolina

EDITOR

ANGELA RICHARD-EAGLIN, DNP, MSN, APRN, FNP-BC, CNE, FAANP, CDE
Associate Dean for Equity, Associate Clinical Professor, Yale School of Nursing, Orange, Connecticut

AUTHORS

ANDREA M. ALEXIS, DNP, APRN, MHA
Veteran Affairs Nursing Academic Partnership (VANAP) Co-Director, Atlanta VA Health Care System, Nursing Education, Decatur, Georgia

JEMMA AYVAZIAN, DNP, ANP-BC, AOCNP, PMGT-BC, FAANP, FAAN
Director of Nursing Education, Office of Academic Affiliations, US Department of Veterans Affairs, Washington, DC

KENYA V. BEARD, EdD, AGACNP-BC, CNE, ANEF, FAAN
Associate Provost Social Mission and Academic Excellence, Chamberlain University, Chicago, Illinois

LYN BEHNKE, DNP, FNP-BC, PMHNP-BC, CAFCI, CTEL, CHFN
Assistant Professor of Nursing, School of Nursing, University of Michigan–Flint, Flint, Michigan

SHERLEY BELIZAIRE, DNP, PMHNP-BC, FNP-BC
Psychiatric-Mental Health Nurse Practitioner and Director, Mental Health Nurse Practitioner Residency Program, US Department of Veteran Affairs, VA Boston Healthcare System, Brockton, Massachusetts

LACRECIA M. BELL, MSN, RN
Clinical Nurse Educator, Duke University School of Nursing, Durham, North Carolina

KEISHA BELLAMY, MSN, MBA, NE-BC
San Francisco VA Health Care System, San Francisco, California

SUSAN BRASHER, PhD, RN, CPNP-PC, FAAN
Assistant Professor, Tenure Track, Nell Hodgson Woodruff School of Nursing, Emory University, Atlanta, Georgia

LISA BURKHART, PhD, RN, ANEF
Research Health Scientist, Center of Innovation for Complex Chronic Healthcare, Edward Hines, Jr. VA Hospital, US Department of Veterans Affairs, Hines, Illinois; Associate Professor, Marcella Niehoff School of Nursing, Loyola University Chicago, Chicago, Illinois

MARY E. DESMOND, PhD, RN, AHN-BC
Research Health Scientist, Center of Innovation for Complex Chronic Healthcare, Edward Hines, Jr. VA Hospital, US Department of Veterans Affairs, Hines, Illinois; Associate Director, Master's Entry to Nursing Practice Program, DePaul University, Chicago, Illinois

ALEXIS DICKINSON, PMHNP-BC
US Department of Veteran Affairs, VA Boston Healthcare System, Brockton, Massachusetts

KATHARINA V. ECHT, PhD
Associate Director Education and Evaluation, Birmingham/Atlanta VA Geriatric Research Education and Clinical Center (GRECC), Atlanta VA Health Care System, Brookhaven, Georgia; Associate Professor of Medicine, Division of Geriatrics and Gerontology, Emory University School of Medicine, Atlanta, Georgia

IRENE C. FELSMAN, DNP, MPH, RN
Assistant Professor, Duke University School of Nursing, Duke Global Health Institute, Durham, North Carolina

SELENA GILLES, DNP, ANP-BC, CNEcl, FNYAM
Associate Dean, Undergraduate Program, Clinical Associate Professor, New York University, Rory Meyers College of Nursing, New York, New York

BEVERLY GONZALEZ, PhD
Statistician, Center of Innovation for Complex Chronic Healthcare, Edward Hines, Jr. VA Hospital, US Department of Veterans Affairs, Hines, Illinois

ROSA M. GONZALEZ-GUARDA, PhD, MPH, RN, CPH, FAAN
Associate Professor, Duke University School of Nursing, Duke Clinical Translational Science Institute, Durham, North Carolina

STEPHANIE N.S. HOSLEY, DNP, APRN-CNP, CNE
Assistant Professor of Clinical Practice, Pediatric Nurse Practitioner Specialty Track Director, College of Nursing, The Ohio State University, Columbus, Ohio

ROSIE JONES, MS
Management Analyst, Office of Academic Affiliations, US Department of Veterans Affairs, Washington, DC

WRENETHA A. JULION, PhD, MPH, RN, CNL, FAAN
Professor and Associate Dean for Equity and Inclusion, Rush University, Chicago, Illinois

TRACIE WALKER KIRKLAND, DNP, ANP-BC, CPNP
Clinical Associate Professor, Department of Nursing, University of Southern California, Suzanne Dworak-Peck School of Social Work, Texas Women's University, PhD Student, Los Angeles, California

MICHAEL L. MCFARLAND, DNP, AGACNP-BC, FNP-BC
Lead APP, Division of Hospital Medicine, Emory Midtown, Clinical Instructor, Emory University, Nell Hodgson Woodruff School of Nursing, Atlanta, Georgia

JACQUELYN McMILLIAN-BOHLER, PhD, CNM, CNE
Assistant Professor, Duke University School of Nursing, Durham, North Carolina

KATERINA MELINO, MS, PMHNP-BC
Co-Director, Psychiatric Mental Health Nurse Practitioner Program, Assistant Clinical Professor, UCSF School of Nursing, San Francisco, California

ANNA MIRK, MD
Associate Director Clinical Innovation, Birmingham/Atlanta VA Geriatric Research Education and Clinical Center (GRECC), Atlanta VA Health Care System, Brookhaven, Georgia; Associate Professor of Medicine, Division of Geriatrics and Gerontology, Emory University School of Medicine, Atlanta, Georgia

LISA MUIRHEAD, DNP, APRN, ANP-BC, FAANP, FAAN
Associate Professor Clinical Track, Associate Dean for Equity and Inclusion, Admissions, and Student Affairs, Emory University, Nell Hodgson Woodruff School of Nursing, Atlanta, Georgia

ANGELA RICHARD-EAGLIN, DNP, MSN, APRN, FNP-BC, CNE, FAANP, CDE
Associate Dean for Equity, Associate Clinical Professor, Yale School of Nursing, Orange, Connecticut

ROSA M. SOLORZANO, MPH, MD
Consulting Associate, Duke University School of Nursing, Duke University Romance Studies SLP, Durham, North Carolina

JENNIFER L. STAPEL-WAX, PsyD
Associate Professor, Division of Autism and Related Disorders, Department of Pediatrics, Emory University School of Medicine, Director, Infant Toddler Clinical Research Operations, Director, Infant Toddler Community Outreach Research Core, Marcus Autism Center, Children's Healthcare of Atlanta, Atlanta, Georgia USA

ANNA STREWLER, MS, AGPCNP-BC
Assistant Clinical Professor, San Francisco VA Health Care System, University of California, San Francisco, San Francisco, California

ROBERTA WAITE, EdD, PMHCNS, ANEF, FAAN
Professor and Dean Select, Drexel University, Philadelphia, Pennsylvania

MICHELLE WEBB, DNP, RN, BC-CHPCA
Clinical Assistant Professor, Duke University School of Nursing, Durham, North Carolina

JENNIFER WOO, PhD, CNM/WHNP, FACNM
Assistant Professor, Texas Woman's University, T. Boone Pickens Institute of Health Sciences, College of Nursing, Dallas, Texas

Contents

Foreword: Addressing and Dismantling Inequities of Vulnerable Populations **xiii**

Benjamin Smallheer

Preface: Vulnerable Populations: Erasing the Margins to Advance Health Equity **xv**

Angela Richard-Eaglin

Challenges to Telehealth: What Was Learned from Families of Children with Neurodevelopmental Disorders **315**

Stephanie N.S. Hosley

Children with neurodevelopmental disorders (NDD) are a vulnerable population diagnosed as having an impairment of the central nervous system caused by genetic, metabolic, toxic or traumatic factors. During the coronavirus disease 2019 (COVID-19) pandemic children with NDD benefitted from the swift transition to telehealth. Most found telehealth favorable but some encountered challenges with accessibility and technology. Racial disparity was found with accessibility challenges by marginalized groups within this already vulnerable population. Telehealth use should continue to be utilized by children with NDD but clinicians should be aware of how to address challenges.

Social Determinants of Health: Considerations for Care of Older Veterans **329**

Lisa Muirhead, Katharina V. Echt, Andrea M. Alexis, and Anna Mirk

Social determinants of health (SDOH), the environments and circumstances in which people are born, grow, live, work and age, are potent drivers of health, health disparities, and health outcomes over the lifespan. Military service affords unique experiences, exposures, and social and health vulnerabilities which impact the life course and may alter health equity and health outcomes for older veterans. Identifying and addressing SDOH, inclusive of the military experience, allows person-centered, more equitable care to this vulnerable population. Nurses and other health professionals should be familiar with how to identify and address health-related social needs and implement interdiciplinary, team-based approaches to connect patients with resources and benefits specifically available to veterans.

Identifying Suicide Risk Factors in Lesbian, Gay, Bisexual, Transgender, and Queer Veterans **347**

Sherley Belizaire, Alexis Dickinson, and Michelle Webb

The purpose of this article is to provide an overview of risk and protective factors for suicide in the lesbian (L), gay (G), bisexual (B), transgender (T), and queer (Q) veteran population, identify the tools and resources necessary to address their mental health needs and outline an evidence-based approach for community health care professionals to use as a guide for treatment and suicide prevention in this unique population. The importance of applying an intersectional lens to the multidimensional identity of LGTQ veterans is emphasized. Recommendations are provided for safety planning, follow-up, and treatment.

Caring for Veteran Women: Collaborative Nursing Approaches to Improve Care **359**

Anna Strewler and Keisha Bellamy

A strength-based nursing approach to recommendations for interpersonal collaboration and communication is used when caring for Veteran women in health care settings. Four areas are emphasized: (1) using trauma-informed health care practices; (2) acknowledging and affirming the intersectional identities of Veteran women to individualize care and counteract health disparities; (3) engaging strategies to enhance a sense of belonging for Veteran women in health care settings; and (4) encouraging Veteran women to participate in potential research studies to better understand and improve care for this population.

US Department of Veterans Affairs Post-Baccalaureate Registered Nurse Residency: Developing Nurses Equipped with Knowledge and Skills to Care for Nation's Veterans **375**

Jemma Ayvazian, Beverly Gonzalez, Mary E. Desmond, Rosie Jones, and Lisa Burkhart

Nurse residency programs were developed to improve novice nurse competencies, mitigate burnout, lower recruitment costs and nurse attrition, and the quality of patient care. The Office of Academic Affiliations (OAA), US Department of Veterans Affairs (VA), established a 12-month postbaccalaureate nurse residency (PB-RNR) program at 49 sites to develop competent, confident, practice-ready registered nurses equipped with the knowledge and skills to care for veterans. The OAA evaluation of the PB-RNR program demonstrated improved new nurse graduate competence, confidence, recruitment, and retention rates after completion of training at participating VA medical facilities.

Promoting Health Equity in the Latinx Community, Locally and Globally: The Duke University School of Nursing Model **393**

Rosa M. Gonzalez-Guarda, Irene C. Felsman, and Rosa M. Solorzano

It is imperative that nurses are equipped to promote the health and well-being of diverse populations in United States, including the growing Latinx community, which experiences significant health disparities. This article summarizes the values, programs, and impact of the Duke University School of Nursing Latinx Engagement Health Equity Model. Collaborative partnerships with diverse community partners addressing Latinx populations across the life span were developed, spanning the education, research, and service missions of the university. Programs were rooted in cultural values and were delivered through diverse interprofessional teams and with support from the university. Programs included local and global immersion programs, volunteer work, courses in Medical Spanish, community engaged research projects, and leadership in coalitions. These models have resulted in favorable outcomes for learners, faculty and staff, and the Latinx community more broadly and can serve as a model for strategies to promote health equity at schools of nursing.

Rural and Indigenous Vulnerable Populations: A Case Study **413**

Lyn Behnke

This is an actual case study of a young Native American man. The names have changed but the challenges remain the same. The intersectionality between the Native population, a rural community, and poverty intersects to create a compelling look at the challenges people face in these communities. Implications for Nursing in relation to practice, education, and policy are addressed.

Applying Cultural Intelligence to Improve Vaccine Hesitancy Among Black, Indigenous, and People of Color **421**

Angela Richard-Eaglin and Michael L. McFarland

Despite the overwhelming evidence to support the benefits of vaccines for preventable diseases and improving health outcomes throughout the world, vaccine hesitancy and resistance continues to be a concern during the COVID-19 pandemic. Although Black, Indigenous, and People of Color (BIPOC) experience the highest rates of morbidity and mortality from COVID-19, mistrust and historical unethical research and medical practices continue to preclude this population from getting the vaccine. This article urges clinicians to subscribe to development and application of cultural intelligence to understand the impact of structural racism and cultural considerations of BIPOC to partner in strategy development.

Structural Competency in Health Care **433**

Katerina Melino

The pandemics of COVID-19, systemic racism, and accelerating climate crises that have unfolded over the last 2 years highlight how social structures bear significant and disparate effects on individual health. The framework of structural competency offers a new way to understand and respond to health inequities in clinical care and health services delivery. Clinicians can work toward achieving structural competency at the individual, interpersonal, clinic, and community levels using the interventions described in the article.

Considerations and Recommendations for Care of Black Pregnant Patients During COVID-19 **443**

Jacquelyn McMillian-Bohler and Lacrecia M. Bell

Black pregnant patients experience perinatal morbidity and mortality rates greater than other ethnic groups. These health disparities exist primarily because of systemic racism, bias, and discriminatory acts within the health care system. The COVID-19 pandemic has reinforced health disparities experienced by all vulnerable populations in the United States, including black pregnant patients. This article highlights some of the factors that may impact the experience of black people as they navigate the COVID-19 pandemic and presents strategies that every provider can implement to minimize the detrimental effects of this devastating virus during pregnancy.

Educators Countering the Impact of Structural Racism on Health Equity **453**

Kenya V. Beard, Wrenetha A. Julion, and Roberta Waite

Health equity endorses that all persons are respected equally, and society must exert intentional efforts to eradicate inequities. Race, frequently taught as an impartial risk factor for disease, is a facilitator of structural inequities stemming from racist policies. Nursing educators must help students understand the impact of structural racism on patient populations, communities, and society at large. This article illustrates the face of structural racism, highlights how structural racism impacts health care outcomes, and provides meaningful ways for educators to unmute racism and facilitate race-related discourse in the classroom to counter the impact of structural racism on health equity.

Social Support and Loneliness Among Black and Hispanic Senior Women Experiencing Food Insecurity: The Nurse as Primary, Secondary, and Tertiary Intervention **461**

Tracie Walker Kirkland and Jennifer Woo

The impact of social determinants of health (SDOH) is understudied and until recently not a focal point in nursing education. The new Essentials coupled with the impact of the coronavirus (COVID-19) pandemic deem it necessary to address the intersection of SDOH and population health. The impact of COVID 19 disproportionately affects Black and Hispanic families. Couple the disproportionate numbers of COVID 19 among these groups with the growing incidence of food insecurity, and there is a need to explore intersecting links. Emerging research link the lack of social support systems and loneliness to food insecurity. In alignment with addressing competency-based education, it is critical to assess factors such as social support systems and loneliness and the intersection of its effects on such determinants as food insecurity. The article provides an overview for its readers in examining the incidence of food insecurity in older ethnic minority women along with postulated social attributes as contributing factors to the growth rates of food insecurity. The incidence of food insecurity among older ethnic minority women has grown exponentially amid the pandemic. The authors illustrate the role nurses can play in addressing primary, secondary, and tertiary interventions using Neuman's Theory. The intervention pathways are delineated through the lens of nursing theoretic framework created by Betty Neuman Systems Model.

Opioid Overdose Harm Prevention: The Role of the Nurse in Patient Education **477**

Selena Gilles

Opioid overdose continues to affect thousands each year in the United States, with nearly 850,000 lives lost within the last 20 years. It will take a comprehensive and coordinated approach from all members of the health care team and health care institutions, in addition to governmental officials, public safety, and community organizations to mitigate this crisis. Nurses can be instrumental in educating patients, families, and community members about ways to combat this epidemic, instrumental in advocating for their patients, advocating for reform, as well as continuing to bring awareness to this health crisis and provoke dialogue about ongoing solutions to end it.

Racial and Ethnic Disparities in Autism Spectrum Disorder: Implications for Care **489**

Susan Brasher, Jennifer L. Stapel-Wax, and Lisa Muirhead

Autism spectrum disorder (ASD) is a complex neurodevelopmental disorder characterized by difficulties with social interaction and communication and the presence of restrictive and repetitive behavior. Individuals with ASD, particularly those from diverse racial and ethnic backgrounds, are at higher risk of certain health conditions and mortality over the lifespan. Disparities in timing of diagnosis, access to services, and quality of care have a significant impact on the trajectory of individuals on the autism spectrum. Health care providers and law enforcement officers often interact with individuals with ASD and need adequate preparation to provide person-centered care to this vulnerable population.

NURSING CLINICS

FORTHCOMING ISSUES

December 2022
The Future of Nursing: Advancing Nursing Education and Practice Through Technology
Joni Tornwall, *Editor*

March 2023
COVID-19 and Pandemic Preparedness: Lessons Learned and Next Steps
Kelly A. Wolgast, *Editor*

June 2023
Substance Use and Abuse
Linda Stone, *Editor*

RECENT ISSUES

June 2022
Nursing Leadership in Long-Term Care
Melodee Harris, Ann Kolanowski, and Sherry Greenberg, *Editors*

March 2022
Burnout in Nursing: Causes, Management, and Future Directions
George A. Zangaro, Dorothy Dulko, Debra Sullivan, *Editors*

December 2021
Obesity
Angela Golden, *Editor*

Foreword

Addressing and Dismantling Inequities of Vulnerable Populations

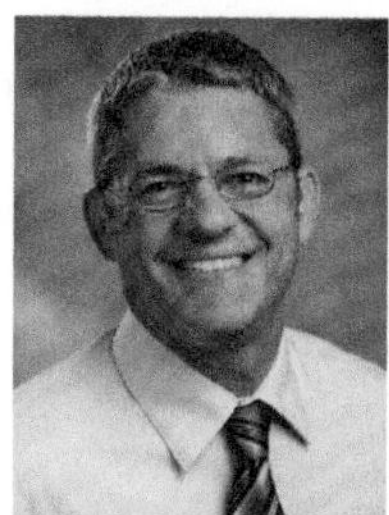

Benjamin Smallheer, PhD, RN, ACNP-BC, FNP-BC, CCRN, CNE
Consulting Editor

Health care in the United States continues efforts to dismantle a system that disadvantages those from vulnerable and marginalized populations. *Healthy People 2030* aims to improve health and well-being over the next decade with attention to health conditions, health behaviors, populations, settings and systems, and social determinants of health that impact at-risk groups. Health equity, health literacy, and social determinants of health are priority areas of concern for the US Department of Health and Human Services.[1] This essential work cannot be fully advanced without first asking a fundamental question: Who are the populations at risk? Are they vulnerable populations, marginalized populations, disadvantaged populations, and what does the use of such qualifiers insinuate?

Vulnerable populations are identified as those at risk for poor physical, psychological, or social health.[2] Factors that either place or contribute to a higher risk of vulnerability include, but are not limited to, belonging to communities of color, sexual/gender minorities, veterans, individuals with substance dependence, individuals with psychiatric and mental health needs, and the intersectionality of any of these. Vulnerable may also suggest the need for protection due to being powerless and helpless to situations or circumstances. These labels can lead to bias, stigmatization, and exclusion from communities or resources. What is being suggested is that vulnerable populations are individuals or groups at increased risk of harm. Working toward improved outcomes relies on a more thoughtful discussion of populations who are at greater risk with a goal of enhancing knowledge and understanding, and eventually improved patient care. There is a chance, however, of implicit bias when referring to an individual or group as "vulnerable." If we accept the premise of vulnerable populations, does that then suggest, and are we accepting, that invulnerable populations also exist?[3]

Nurs Clin N Am 57 (2022) xiii–xiv
https://doi.org/10.1016/j.cnur.2022.07.001
0029-6465/22/© 2022 Published by Elsevier Inc.

We must intentionally direct attention to consider the factors that put individuals and populations "at risk" and question what has led to a system where inequitable health care exists. This issue of *Nursing Clinics of North America* expands our knowledge and understanding of caring for vulnerable, underserved, and marginalized people and communities. We draw attention to our communities of color, sexual/gender minorities, veterans, individuals with substance dependence, and individuals with psychiatric and mental health needs…while also recognizing this is not an all-encompassing list. We must be intentional in our care…and the time is now for these intentional acts.

Benjamin Smallheer, PhD, RN, ACNP-BC, FNP-BC, CCRN, CNE
Duke University
School of Nursing
307 Trent Drive
Box 3322, Office 3117
Durham, NC 27710, USA

E-mail address:
benjamin.smallheer@duke.edu

REFERENCES

1. Office of Disease Prevention and Health Promotion. Diabetes. Healthy people 2030. US Department of Health and Human Services. Available at: https://health.gov/healthypeople. Accessed June 29, 2022.
2. Webber-Ritchey KJ, Simonovich SD, Spurlark RS. COVID-19: qualitative research with vulnerable populations. Nurs Sci Q 2021;34(1):13–9. https://doi.org/10.1177/0894318420965225.
3. Munari SC, Wilson AN, Blow NJ, et al. Rethinking the use of 'vulnerable. Aust N Z Public Health 2021;45(3):197–9.

Preface

Vulnerable Populations: Erasing the Margins to Advance Health Equity

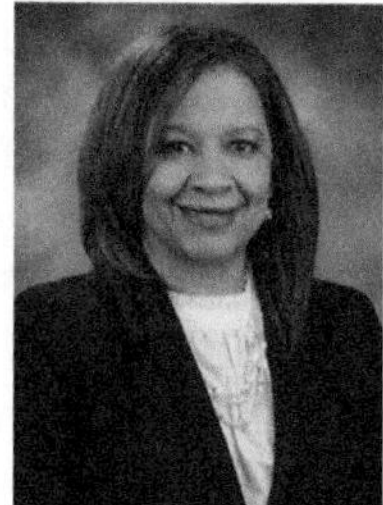

Angela Richard-Eaglin, DNP, MSN, APRN, FNP-BC, CNE, FAANP, CDE
Editor

For the last three decades, the US Department of Health and Human Services Office of Disease Prevention and Health Promotion has issued 10-year objectives for improving health and well-being. Each iteration has specific foci that includes measurable goals. At the culmination of each 10-year decade, progress is evaluated, and the findings from previous decades are used to build upon lessons learned and apply that information to ongoing *Healthy People* efforts. The most current iteration, *Healthy People 2030*, released in 2020, includes a more amplified focus on health equity, *Social Determinants of Health* (SDOH), health literacy, and well-being. The topics of vulnerable populations, health inequities, and the SDOH are integral for transforming health care systems and health care delivery. These topics are critical in creating sustainable interventions that support well-being, advance health equity, and eliminate disparities. Health inequities, which are a direct consequence of structural disenfranchisement, have long plagued historically underrepresented, marginalized, and stigmatized individuals and populations. Identifying, acknowledging, and prioritizing individual needs and population health are paramount for substantial positive change in overall health outcomes to happen. Achieving the *Healthy People 2030* mission, "building a healthier future for all," and attaining the SDOH goals can only become a reality with targeted and deliberate interventions aimed at dismantling and restructuring current policies and practices that have consistently and considerably impeded progress.

Vulnerable populations include those with unique health care and survival needs, including support, resources, safeguards, and those at risk of abuse, neglect, or unsafe conditions and outcomes. This description alone should actuate immediate acknowledgment and prioritization of the health care needs of individuals and

Nurs Clin N Am 57 (2022) xv–xvi
https://doi.org/10.1016/j.cnur.2022.06.001
0029-6465/22/© 2022 Published by Elsevier Inc.

communities who are vulnerable. Using the word vulnerable to describe people has been and continues to be a point of contention in some spaces; however, effectuating meaningful interventions that advance health equity requires naming/labeling issues as exactly what they are. Vulnerability is not a negative or derogatory term. The state of being vulnerable is resultant from inherent or external factors beyond individual control. Clinicians may not routinely consider the additional circumstances and conditions that compound and further compromise health outcomes for susceptible individuals. Therefore, vulnerability is a term that health care professionals should recognize as a prompt to explore additional needs requirements and development of individualized, holistic, and culturally responsible plans of care for individuals and populations.

Advancing health equity to achieve health optimal outcomes requires dissemination of information, strategies, and interventions specific to vulnerable populations that health care providers can apply in academic and clinical settings. This issue of *Nursing Clinics of North America* covers a broad spectrum of considerations that may be overlooked when caring for vulnerable, underserved, and marginalized people and communities.

Angela Richard-Eaglin, DNP, MSN, APRN, FNP-BC, CNE, FAANP, CDE
Yale School of Nursing
400 West Campus Drive
Orange, CT 06516-0972, USA

1326 Chariot Drive
Baton Rouge, LA 70816, USA

E-mail addresses:
angela.richard-eaglin@yale.edu; eaglinagela@gmail.com

Challenges to Telehealth

What Was Learned from Families of Children with Neurodevelopmental Disorders

Stephanie N.S. Hosley, DNP, APRN-CNP, CNE*

KEYWORDS

- Neurodevelopmental disorders • Telehealth
- Children with neurodevelopmental disorders • Telehealth in vulnerable populations

KEY POINTS

- Telehealth visits have provided a safe alternative to in-person visits during the COVID-19 pandemic.
- Children with neurodevelopmental disorders can benefit from telehealth utilization but may experience some challenges.
- Racial disparities exist in telehealth accessibility.

Abbreviations	
NDD	neurodevelopmental disorders

INTRODUCTION

Coronavirus disease 2019(COVID-19) has affected all facets of life since its beginning. Healthcare delivery has not escaped the impact. Hospital and clinician shift to limit exposure and utilize limited resources acted as a springboard for rapid growth of telehealth utilization. One source reports an increase of 2938% since the start of the pandemic.[1] The increase has brought both benefit and barriers to care. Efficient, evidence-based care is important to maximize health outcomes in any situation. Although telehealth is not a new phenomenon, the data to support evidence-based telehealth care to reduce the barriers is not widely available.

This article will examine the challenges to telehealth as experienced by children with neurodevelopmental disorder (NDD) and their families. The children were all patients at a pediatric hospital in the United States during the first year of the pandemic. It will also provide recommendations for providing equitable care through telehealth to this vulnerable population.

College of Nursing, The Ohio State University, 1585 Neil Avenue, Columbus, OH 43210, USA
* Corresponding author.
E-mail address: Hosley.8@osu.edu

Nurs Clin N Am 57 (2022) 315–328
https://doi.org/10.1016/j.cnur.2022.04.001

HISTORY

In a metropolitan hospital serving the pediatric population, COVID brought changes familiar to other healthcare facilities worldwide. Elective procedures were canceled. Preventative care was rescheduled. And in person visits were significantly reduced to those deemed necessary.

The divisions of the hospital serving children with NDD were impacted by the shift. For families of children with NDD challenges with canceled and rescheduled appointments was just a start. Home health nursing was limited in many cases to reduce risk of exposure. Therapeutic services including physical, occupational and speech therapy were placed on hold. When telehealth became available, for many it may have been viewed as an additional challenge to navigate.

Legislation at the federal and state levels supported expansion of telehealth services through policy change on allowable providers, location and reimbursement.[2] Within a 2-month period the shift to utilize telehealth visits in many clinics was carefully and rapidly rolled out in an attempt to meet the healthcare needs of its patients. As reliance on telehealth increased, patient feedback was needed for future planning.

BACKGROUND

Children with Neurodevelopmental Disorder

Children with neurodevelopmental disorders (NDD) are diagnosed as having an impairment of the central nervous system caused by genetic, metabolic, toxic or traumatic factors.[3] Common diagnoses include cerebral palsy, autism spectrum disorder, Down Syndrome, traumatic brain injury and multiple genetic syndromes. Children with NDD frequently have multiple diagnoses and are dependent on medical technology for some component of their lives. This technology could include nutrition, respiratory or ambulatory support.

Children with NDD have varying levels of cognitive ability. Many have limited to no verbal communication skills. These children may ambulate independently or rely on assistive devices to move around.

This population requires care by an interdisciplinary team that may include therapists, advanced practice registered nurses, physician assistants, physicians and social workers. This team is in addition to the team of teachers and support personnel that address their medical needs during the school day. Well-rounded care of these children results in not only increased monetary cost, but indirect costs related to the time involved.

Children with NDD represent less than 2% of the children in the United States. Yet costs related to their care has been documented to be as high as 143% of costs related to typically developing children vastly outweighing the medical costs for the other 98% of US children.[4] It is imperative that clinicians provide quality care while remaining efficient stewards of healthcare resources.

Caregiver Stress

Parents of children with NDD transport their children to multiple appointments on a routine basis. This necessitates the caregiver juggle the schedule of the child with NDD and often that of other children, family members, as well as their own employment requirements. A study by Bentenuto and colleagues demonstrated the increased stress levels experienced by parents of children with NDD before and during the pandemic.[5] Stress can emanate from care, lost sleep, financial burden, lack of social and emotional support and job performance.[6]

As previously stated, families of children with NDD report a higher level of stress than parents of neurotypical children at baseline. Concern existed for the impact of COVID-19 to magnify that stress. A scoping review examined the challenges caused by COVID-19 for families of children with NDD. The resulting themes included challenges with behavioral issues, disruption of daily activity and challenges with existing resources to assist families.[7]

Children with NDD have varying levels of dependence on caregivers throughout the day. Some are dependent on others for all activities related to daily living. During the pandemic, families balanced COVID-19 exposure risk against shouldering the care previously shared by a team of family and paid providers. Families closed their doors to people outside their home to maintain safety. Some studies indicated the isolation and increased care burden experienced by the families not only increased parental stress but had a negative impact on behaviors of the children.[7,8]

Education was also negatively impacted. The patients and families lacked the support, training and knowledge available in the schools to help their children accomplish their schoolbased tasks.[9] Pasca and colleagues demonstrated almost 40% of patients in a study reported challenges with completing schoolwork.[9] Parents were acting in the role of parent, nurse, aide and teacher. With the increased workload they were unable to adhere to the child's routine schedule. This impact of the disruption in routine was demonstrated by some with an increase in disruptive behavior. It was also demonstrated in some with a decrease in family functioning.[10]

Telehealth

Telehealth is defined as the use of electronic information and telecommunications technology to provide care from a distance. Telehealth delivery can vary and can include both audio-only and combined audio-video visits.[11,12] Telehealth was first recorded in the early 20th century when data was transmitted via the telephone wires.[13] It advanced gradually each decade and then exploded during the pandemic.[13]

Telehealth can be used to deliver routine and episodic care through a variety of mechanisms including tablets, computers, and telephones. Telehealth has been provided through both 1:1 and in a hub and spoke format. In the hub and spoke format, a patient goes to a physical location managed by a technician or other member of the health care team. The team member may utilize equipment that transmits information or images to a clinician at a satellite location or hub. This enables the patient to be seen by a specialist whose distance or schedule prohibits an in-person visit.

Telehealth and the Impact on Children with Neurodevelopmental Disorders

During the pandemic the use of telehealth decreased potential exposure of the patient and healthcare staff to COVID-19. Caregivers of children with NDD avoided the arduous process of transporting a nonambulatory child and the necessary lifesaving equipment such as portable ventilators and wheelchairs. When possible this was replaced with use of an electronic device to engage with their healthcare team, saving time and travel related expenses.

Published studies on telehealth use during the pandemic have reported up to 70% of parents of children with NDD used telehealth during the pandemic.[14] In the same study, nearly 50% of those surveyed reported overall satisfaction. Only 30% thought the services worked well for their children.[14] Details on the discrepancy between overall satisfaction and what worked well were not available.

Telehealth benefits were observed by clinicians caring for patients with NDD. The Society for Developmental & Behavioral Pediatrics cited improved access, increased naturalistic observations, reduced travel challenges and cost reduction as reasons supporting telehealth.[15] Children with NDD can experience increased stress when in unfamiliar environments. Clinician ability to observe patients in their homes through telehealth offered a different perspective to develop a diagnosis and resulting plan of care. Tools have been and continue to be developed and validated to improve the diagnostic process via telehealth.[16]

Caregivers also reported benefits related to telehealth utilization. Families noted the improvement in travel time and decreased fuel costs avoided with telehealth. A study demonstrated 30% of families reported a time savings of over 3 hours related to reduced travel with telehealth.[17] Caregivers also reported appreciation that some services were able to continue via telehealth, avoiding a regression in skills.[18]

Benefits to telehealth could also serve a dual role as a barrier. A child's familiarity with their home surroundings sometimes contributed to distractibility and interfered with engagement during the exam.[16] Telehealth visits also lacked the hands-on assessment needed to properly diagnose causes of change in function or discomfort. Challenges exist in assessing some children with NDD secondary to inability to assess muscle tone and coordination.[12]

Parents reported concern that the online environment impacted the child's ability to engage. Additionally, caregivers reported challenges with multitasking during the appointments related to managing care of multiple children in the home.[18] Some therapy sessions were beyond what a single caregiver at home could manage. A single adult in the home would have challenges positioning the child while also trying to adjust the camera.[19] The literature also discusses caregivers experience of challenges accessing technology.[17]

Broadband Access

Current estimates on U.S. households lacking access to high-quality broadband varies widely between 19 million to 42 million.[12,20] Correlations between household access to an electronic device and household income have been documented.[20] Families experiencing increased stress and decreased resources during the pandemic may not have had the ability to access a device and/or internet access to facilitate a telehealth visit. There were multiple reports of families driving to a local school or library to access Wi-Fi from the parking lot.

Historically, marginalized populations disproportionately lack access to broadband either through internet access itself or access to a useable device. According to 2015 US Census data Black households were least likely to own all types of electronic devices and/or have broadband access.[20] Marginalized groups were also more likely to only have access to handheld devices verses a tablet or laptop computer.[20]

METHODS

Context

A survey requesting patient feedback on telehealth was developed and distributed through email following their telehealth visit. Data on patient perspectives of challenges with telehealth was deemed important in quality improvement related to telehealth. The survey consisted of 30 questions on general experience and ease of scheduling, care provided by staff and challenges related to use of telehealth. Information on gender, race, ethnicity, geographic location, provider type, primary diagnosis, language, interpreter use and reason for visit were captured.

Ethical Considerations

Division specific data was distributed automatically to management. The author requested and received IRB approval to review the data specific to patients with NDD. The study was deemed exempt.

Measures

The survey used a Likert scale of 1 to 5 to indicate respondents' level of agreement with a particular statement. Zeroes were used to indicate a response was unchecked to a specific question, despite answering others. Dashes were used to record lack of response to a specific record.

The survey questions related to perceived challenges to use of telehealth can be grouped into five categories. The categories are listed in **Table 1**. It also provides a list of the questions on perceived challenges.

Although the survey was used hospital wide, this discussion focuses on the responses by clinics primarily serving the needs of children with NDD including a clinic focused on managing developmental behavioral pediatrics, the interdisciplinary cerebral palsy team and a complex healthcare clinic that serves as a primary care home for children with NDD. The responses were collected over a 6-month period.

Table 1
Survey questions on perceived challenges of telehealth

	Perceived Challenges Legend
Accessibility/Technology	
1	Challenges finding internet access
2	Challenges finding a suitable digital device (such as smartphone, tablet, computer)
3	Trouble logging into MyChart
4	Trouble starting the video call (Zoom)
5	Not sure how to carry out a telehealth visit
6	Need for translation services
7	Not able to directly get written records (such as medical record and educational materials)
Comfort/Privacy	
8	Finding a quiet, private place to carry out the visit
9	Not comfortable with physical exposure on camera over the video visit
Quality	
10	Worried about the quality of telehealth visits
Financial	
11	Concerns about whether the visit would be covered by insurance
Other	
12	COVID-19 related impact on scheduling a visit (eg, no childcare, changing work schedule)
13	Concerns about policy
14	Other

RESULTS

Participants

Survey data from a 6-month period of distribution was reviewed. Three hundred ninety-eight responses were received from families and caregivers for children with NDD seen for medical, behavioral, and nutritional needs. Primary diagnoses for the visits included cerebral palsy, attention deficit hyperactivity disorder (ADHD), intellectual disability, constipation, upper respiratory infection, global developmental delay, autism spectrum disorder, avoidant restrictive food intake disorder (ARFID), anxiety, mitochondrial metabolism disorder, trisomy 21, feeding difficulties and disruptive behavior.

Over half of the respondents, left multiple questions unanswered. The email request was the singular opportunity to respond to the survey. There were no in-person or paper surveys offered in the clinic setting. There were no follow-up inquiries based on survey results. **Table 2** lists demographic data.

Over the 6-month period of data collection, 176 (44%) of the visits were completed by physicians, advanced practice registered nurses and psychologists. Most patients with NDD are managed by multidisciplinary teams. Additional clinicians that provided

Table 2
Demographic data of sample (N = 398)

Variable	N (%)
Gender	
Male	288 (72)
Female	110 (28)
Race	
Asian	10 (3)
Black or African American	55 (14)
Multiple Race	37 (9)
Unknown	6 (1)
White	290 (73)
Ethnicity	
Hispanic or Latino	18 (5)
No information	7 (1)
Not Hispanic or Latino	373 (94)
Primary Language	
Arabic	2 (<1)
English	371 (93)
Other	12 (3)
Somali	2 (<1)
Spanish	11 (3)
Age (Years)	
1–3	49 (12)
4–6	60 (15)
7–12	172 (43)
13–18	102 (26)
>19	15 (4)

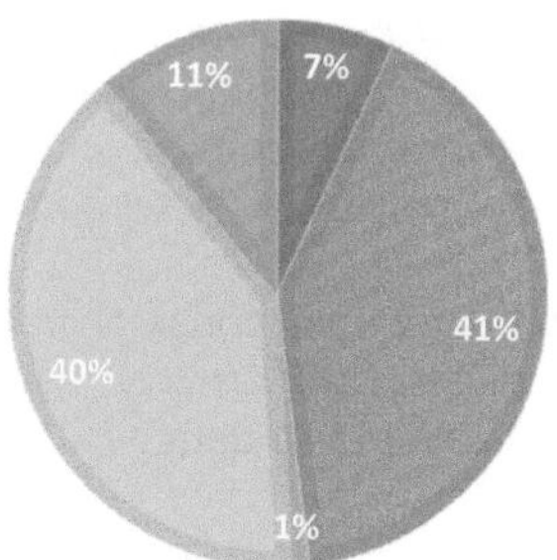

Fig. 1. Count of devices used to access telehealth.

care included social workers, dietitians, behavioral health technicians, therapists, counselors, fellows, and interns. All visits analyzed were completed using the Zoom video conferencing platform to ensure privacy and security; except two that were completed via phone. Reasons explaining the switch to phone from a video visit were not captured in the survey.

Numerous devices were used to complete the visits. Slightly more families reported use of a smartphone than a laptop. Details are provided in **Fig. 1**. Although expansion in reimbursement temporarily allowed for limited use of telephone only visits, the vast majority of visits included audiovisual input.

Challenges to Telehealth

The survey included 17 questions specifically targeted at telehealth use. As many as 58% of respondents left multiple questions unchecked. There were no reported challenges with survey completion recorded in the data set. **Fig. 2** describes the frequency of reported challenges by previously stated categories.

Most reported challenges were accessibility and problems with technology. **Fig. 3** represents results from questions specifically addressing those challenges. When examining the responses in their entirety, challenges with accessing MyChart, the patient portal used to access and begin their visits, was the most reported difficulty. This was followed closely by challenges using the Zoom audiovisual platform.

Differences were noted with some responses when analyzed by race and ethnicity. This analysis was relevant for planning future use of telehealth and addressing Social Determinants of Health. Detailed breakdown for challenges with internet access, finding a suitable device and accessing MyChart are presented in **Figs. 4–6**.

Finding a quiet, private place to carry out the visit was a challenge for 13% of respondents. The exact location of the patient and family during the visit was not captured in the survey. Only 1% of families reported discomfort with physical exposure on camera.

Only 5% of respondents reported concern about insurance coverage of the telehealth visit. Data on patient insurance status was not collected as part of the survey. Neither was insurance type.

Three percent of respondents were concerned about immediate access to written materials. These could include after visit summaries and patient education. All patients using telehealth had MyChart electronic access that may have provided some ability to print educational materials.

Ninety-two percent of respondents agreed that telehealth improved access to healthcare. Of the respondents that did not think access was improved, less than 1% strongly disagreed. Details on why respondents disagreed access was improved was not captured. Data on respondents' opinion on the quality of telehealth to In-Person is detailed in **Fig. 7**. Analysis by provider type followed the trend of the overall group.

Most respondents reported they would consider use of telehealth in the future. **Fig. 8** represents a detailed analysis. Data on why respondents would not use telehealth in the future was not available in this data set.

DISCUSSION

The survey on the telehealth experience was distributed hospital-wide to all patients participating in a telehealth visit. The focus of the author was to examine the challenges experienced by patients and families of children with NDD as they learned to engage with their healthcare team via telehealth. The daily routine of these families is important, and change can result in negative behaviors.[12] Review of the responses revealed 79% had a favorable experience and would agree to use telehealth again.

Challenges were reported more frequently in areas related to accessibility and technology than any other question group. The challenges experienced by this patient population is congruent with that found in the emerging literature.[19] Challenges finding internet access, a suitable device and accessing the patient portal (MyChart) were the most frequent barriers to care reported by the families.

Additionally, concern exists for racial and ethnic disparities in telehealth accessibility based on the responses. Asian respondents reported difficulty with internet access at rates 3 times that of white respondents. Black or African American respondents reported challenges with internet access at twice the rate of white respondents. This is consistent with disparities noted in the literature.[20]

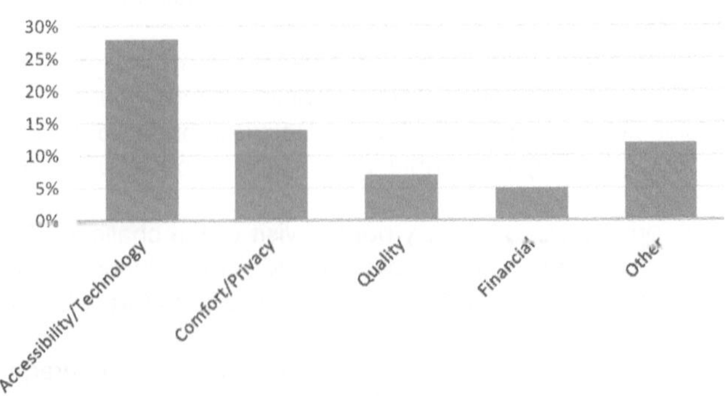

Fig. 2. Challenges by category.

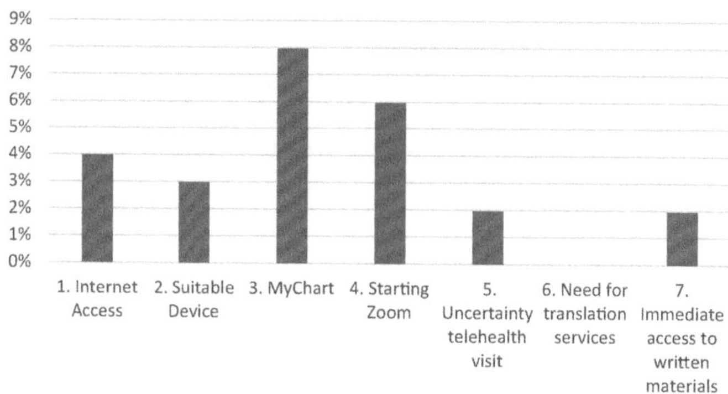

Fig. 3. Challenges to accessibility/technology.

Similar differences were observed in challenges accessing a telehealth suitable device. Seven percent of African Americans agreed they had difficulty accessing a telehealth suitable device. Only 3% of families of white children reported challenges. Zero percent of persons identifying as Asian reported challenges with access to a suitable device. Although the overall percentages of reported difficulties are small, the differences are notable. Fifty percent of African American families reported use of a smartphone to complete the visit. Thirty-nine and 37% respectively of Hispanic and white families reported smartphone use. There was not a question asking the respondent if the handheld device was their only option.

It may be beneficial to develop routine measures to assess broadband access or challenges with telehealth use for persons with multiple recurring appointments. These results reinforce the literature that emphasizes the need to increase access to broadband and suitable devices for children with NDD.[15] Further research is needed on the best way to assess the technology needs.

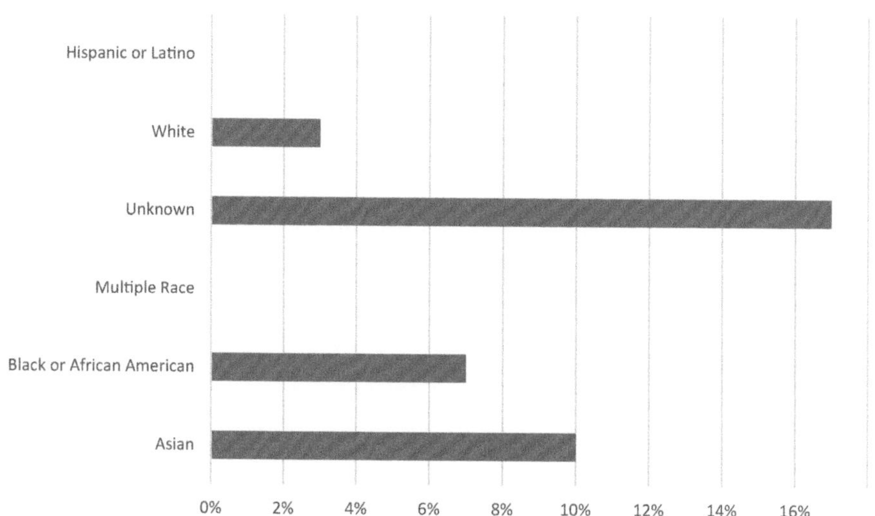

Fig. 4. Challenges with internet access by race and ethnicity.

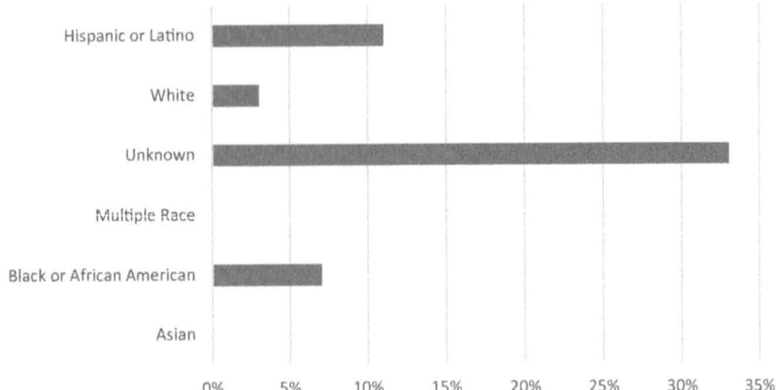

Fig. 5. Challenges with access to a telehealth suitable device by race and ethnicity.

Overall, challenges with MyChart access were the most frequent telehealth challenge identified. This knowledge is important for providers. In many institutions connecting patients and families to resources to assist with access can be done while patients are seen at their in-person visits. The responses for identifying challenges with MyChart varied from other accessibility challenges. Nine percent of white respondents identified challenges with MyChart access while only 5% of black respondents endorsed that accessing MyChart was a challenge.

A total of 18 of respondents had interpretive services scheduled to assist with their video visit. The most frequently assigned was to interpret for those families with an identified hearing loss. This was followed by interpreters for families where Spanish was their primary language. According to the recorded data, only 4 of the families used interpretive services during their telehealth session. It is not known whether the interpreter was not available, the family declined use of interpretive services or if the information on use was omitted in the electronic medical record.

The challenges experienced by the patients in this institution are similar to those discussed in the literature. Also similar to the literature was the overall response from the

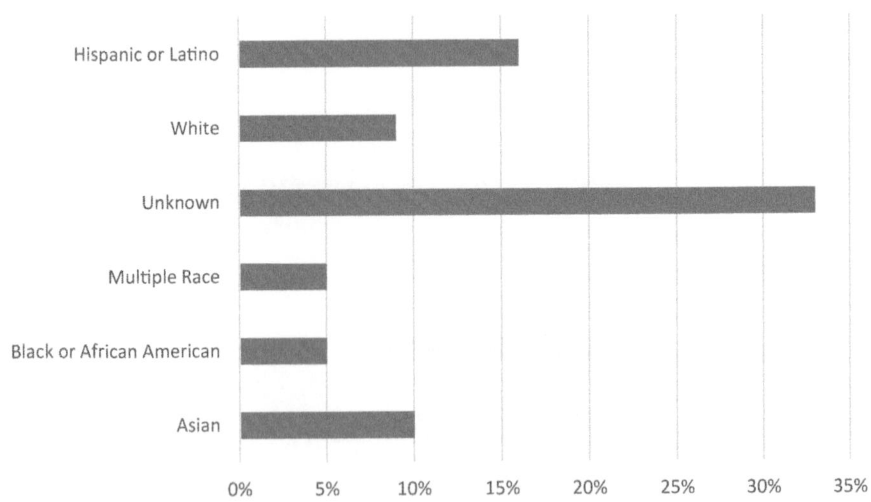

Fig. 6. Challenges logging into MyChart by Race and Ethnicity.

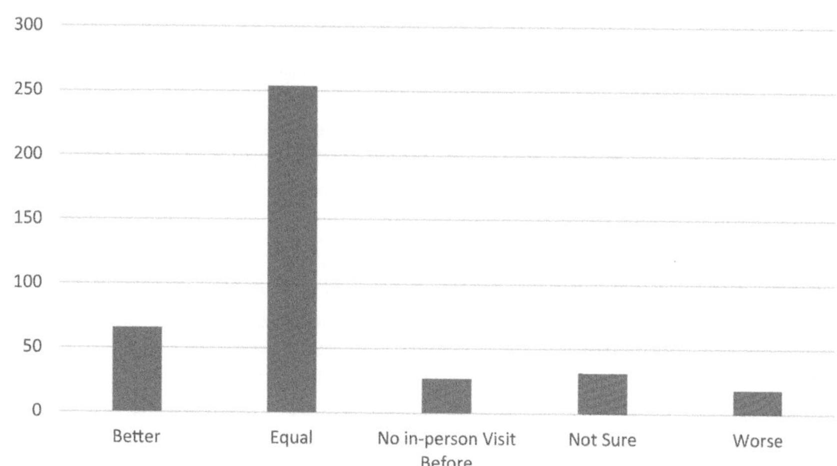

Fig. 7. Count of telehealth compared to in-person visit.

survey respondents as favorable to telehealth use in the future. Telehealth education may need to be a routine component of anticipatory guidance to assist children with NDD and their families with continued telehealth use. Advanced preparation on its purpose and use may decrease accessibility issues. Continued use of telehealth may save families valuable time and money when a telehealth appointment is deemed appropriate for the visit purpose.

LIMITATIONS

An important limitation of this review was the distribution of the survey itself. The survey was sent electronically through email. It is not known if some patients using telehealth were accessing broadband from a location other than their own home. If broadband access was intermittent, the persons experiencing the most challenges may have had limitations in accessing the survey.

Similarly, persons needing interpretive services may have had trouble completing the online survey. This is also true for persons with literacy challenges and may

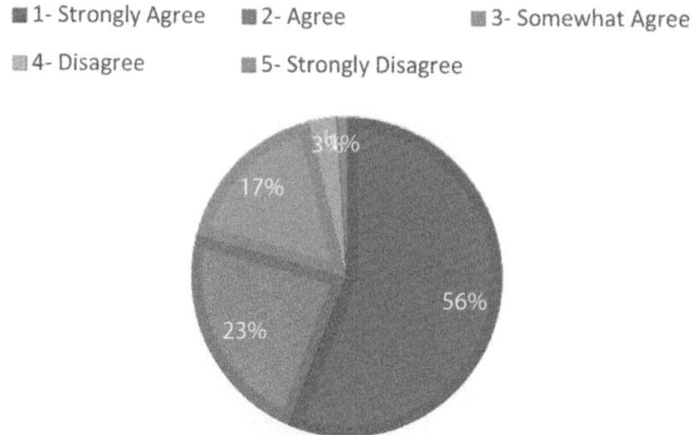

Fig. 8. Family would use video visits in the future.

account for some of the gaps. Connection to interpretive services were made available during the telehealth visit when possible.

The number of incomplete surveys also contributed to the limitations of this project. There were no attempts at in-person completion of surveys secondary to the response to COVID-19. Future projects may utilize both email and in-person completion to capture the responses of those who had difficulty with completion for any reason.

The patients seen in the involved clinics have complex medical needs and represent a small segment of the general pediatric population. The responses from a broader or more homogenous population may yield different results.

SUMMARY

Telehealth use has increased exponentially since the start of the pandemic. For children with complex medical conditions including a neurodevelopmental diagnosis, telehealth provided a safe connection to their frequent healthcare appointments in a time of uncertainty. Telehealth will not disappear as the world transitions from the crisis presented by COVID-19. It is important that clinicians in both clinic-based and hospital settings examine the response from the patients in their community.

The overall response to telehealth in this institution was positive. However, different people will have different experiences. Patients were able to utilize telehealth but experienced some challenges. Ongoing evaluation is needed to improve telehealth models of care and delivery. Increased awareness and understanding of the impact of social determinants of health are also needed to provide equitable, not equal care to this vulnerable population. Use of telehealth will require an evidence-based, team approach to telehealth assessment and to connect patients with resources for success.

CLINICS CARE POINTS

- Use images to assist with communication barriers
- Utilize inclusive intake processes to ask about technology access[21]
- Consider closed captioning options for persons with hearing impairment
- Identify community resources that offer free internet access
- Permit patients to access telehealth from any safe, physical location to decrease barriers to access[15]
- Provide guidance on telehealth visits at an in-person visit

DISCLOSURE

There are no financial conflicts of interest to disclose.

REFERENCES

1. Gelburd R. Telehealth Claim Lines Rise 2938 Percent from November 2019 to November 2020. Am J Manag Care 2021. Available at: https://www-ajmc-com.proxy.lib.ohio-state.edu/view/telehealth-claim-lines-rise-2-938-percent-from-november-2019-to-november-2020.
2. Center for Connected Health Policy. State Telehealth Laws and Medicaid Program Policies Fall 2021. Published online Fall 2021. Available at: https://

www.cchpca.org/2021/10/Fall2021_ExecutiveSummary_FINAL.pdf. Accessed December 30, 2021.

3. Stores G. Multifactorial Influences, Including Comorbidities, Contributing to Sleep Disturbance in Children with a Neurodevelopmental Disorder. CNS Neurosci Ther 2016;22(11):875–9.
4. Lindgren S, Lauer E, Momany E, et al. Disability, Hospital Care, and Cost: Utilization of Emergency and Inpatient Care by a Cohort of Children with Intellectual and Developmental Disabilities. J Pediatr 2021;229:259–66.
5. Bentenuto A, Mazzoni N, Giannotti M, et al. Psychological impact of Covid-19 pandemic in Italian families of children with neurodevelopmental disorders. Res Dev Disabil 2021;109:103840.
6. Rizakos S, Parmar A, Siden HH, et al. The Parental Experience of Caring for a Child With Pain and Irritability of Unknown Origin. J Pain Symptom Manage 2021. https://doi.org/10.1016/j.jpainsymman.2021.07.026.
7. Shorey S, Lau LST, Tan JX, et al. Families With Children With Neurodevelopmental Disorders During COVID-19: A Scoping Review. J Pediatr Psychol 2021;46(5): 514–25.
8. Zhang J, Shuai L, Yu H, et al. Acute stress, behavioural symptoms and mood states among school-age children with attention-deficit/hyperactive disorder during the COVID-19 outbreak. Asian J Psychiatry 2020;51:102077.
9. Pasca L, Zanaboni MP, Grumi S, et al. Impact of COVID-19 pandemic in pediatric patients with epilepsy with neuropsychiatric comorbidities: A telemedicine evaluation. Epilepsy Behav 2021;115:107519.
10. Ehrler M, Werninger I, Schnider B, et al. Impact of the COVID-19 pandemic on children with and without risk for neurodevelopmental impairments. Acta Paediatr 2021;110(4):1281–8.
11. What is telehealth? How is telehealth different from telemedicine? | HealthIT.gov. Available at: https://www.healthit.gov/faq/what-telehealth-how-telehealth-different-telemedicine. Accessed January 1, 2022.
12. Langkamp DL. Has Telehealth Come of Age in Developmental-Behavioral Pediatrics? J Dev Behav Pediatr 2021;42(3):234–5.
13. Wootton R, Geissbuhler A, Jethwani K, et al. Long-running telemedicine networks delivering humanitarian services: experience, performance and scientific output. Bull World Health Organ 2012;90(5):341–347D.
14. Masi A, Mendoza Diaz A, Tully L, et al. Impact of the COVID-19 pandemic on the well-being of children with neurodevelopmental disabilities and their parents. J Paediatr Child Health 2021;57(5):631–6.
15. Keder RD, Mittal S, Stringer K, et al. Society for Developmental & Behavioral Pediatrics Position Statement on Telehealth. J Dev Behav Pediatr 2022;43(1):55–9.
16. Matthews NL, Skepnek E, Mammen MA, et al. Feasibility and acceptability of a telehealth model for autism diagnostic evaluations in children, adolescents, and adults. Autism Res 2021;14(12):2564–79.
17. McNally Keehn R, Enneking B, James C, et al. Telehealth Evaluation of Pediatric Neurodevelopmental Disabilities During the COVID-19 Pandemic: Clinician and Caregiver Perspectives. J Dev Behav Pediatr 2021. https://doi.org/10.1097/DBP.0000000000001043.
18. White SW, Stoppelbein L, Scott H, et al. It took a pandemic: Perspectives on impact, stress, and telehealth from caregivers of people with autism. Res Dev Disabil 2021;113:103938.

19. Wagner L, Corona LL, Weitlauf AS, et al. Use of the TELE-ASD-PEDS for Autism Evaluations in Response to COVID-19: Preliminary Outcomes and Clinician Acceptability. J Autism Dev Disord 2021;51(9):3063–72.
20. Ryan C, Lewis JM. Computer and Internet Use in the United States: 2015. :10.
21. Health Resources & Services Administration. Health equity in telehealth | Telehealth.HHS.gov. Telehealth.HHS.GOV. 2021. Available at: https://telehealth.hhs.gov/providers/health-equity-in-telehealth/. Accessed January 3, 2022.

Social Determinants of Health

Considerations for Care of Older Veterans

Lisa Muirhead, DNP, APRN, ANP-BC, FAANP, FAAN[a,*], Katharina V. Echt, PhD[b,c], Andrea M. Alexis, DNP, APRN, MHA[d], Anna Mirk, MD[b,c]

KEYWORDS

- Veterans • Aged • Social determinants of health • War exposure • Health status • Disparities disparity • Minority and vulnerable populations • Health equity

KEY POINTS

- Social determinants of health (SDOH) are potent drivers of health, health disparities, and health outcomes over the lifespan.
- Military service impacts life course and may alter health equity and health outcomes.
- Older veterans are a vulnerable population with increased risk of health-related problems.
- Identifying and addressing SDOH, including the military experience, are crucial to advance health equity.
- Robust tools and resources exist to address health-related social needs (HRSN) for older veterans.

Social and structural forces that influence health have garnered national attention as these forces, inclusive of socioeconomic status (SES), education, employment, income, and other social determinants significantly contribute to health and health outcomes across the lifespan.[1,2] These social factors are recognized as having greater impact on health than health care, and knowledge of these influencers can inform diagnosis, choices in treatment modalities, health system redesign, and innovation that lend to better health outcomes and lower health care cost.[2] Social factors that drive health disparities among members of marginalized groups are largely attributed to Social determinants of health (SDOH). Understanding the interrelationship and

[a] Emory University, Nell Hodgson Woodruff School of Nursing, 1520 Clifton Road, Atlanta, GA 30322, USA; [b] Veterans Affairs Birmingham/ Atlanta Geriatric Research, Education and Clinical Center (GRECC), Atlanta VA Health Care System, 3101 Clairmont Road Northeast, Brookhaven, GA 30329-1044, USA; [c] Division of Geriatrics and Gerontology, Department of Medicine, Emory University School of Medicine, Atlanta, GA, USA; [d] Atlanta VA Health Care System, Nursing Education, 1M-116A, 1670 Clairmont Road, Decatur, GA 30033, USA
* Corresponding author.
E-mail address: lisa.muirhead@emory.edu

Nurs Clin N Am 57 (2022) 329–345
https://doi.org/10.1016/j.cnur.2022.04.002
0029-6465/22/Published by Elsevier Inc.

complexity of SDOH, nonmedical factors, and the unique life experiences of veterans are vital to providing person-centered, equitable care to our aging veteran population. Here we describe SDOH and their potential protective or adverse influence on health and health outcomes of older veterans given their unique military experiences and exposures. We provide approaches and resources for identifying and addressing health-related social needs (HRSN) of older veterans, a vulnerable population.

SOCIAL DETERMINANTS OF HEALTH AND THEIR SIGNIFICANCE

Social determinants of health (SDOH), defined as the conditions, environments, and circumstances in which people are born, grow, live, work, and age, are potent drivers of health, health risks, health disparities, and health outcomes over time, including in life later.[3–5] The intersectionality of these social factors and economic systems are associated with access to resources that provide protection and maintenance of health. Because inequities in accessing health resources among populations create disparities in health care utilization, morbidity, and mortality, practice-based priorities that focus on recognizing and addressing social needs in health care settings are needed to support clinical decision making.[5–10] The World Health Organization (WHO) purports that SDOH may play a more significant role in health than health care or lifestyle choices, and SDOH can serve to impact health equity adversely or positively.[6] *Healthy People 2030* and the Robert Wood Johnson Foundation indicate that not only do SDOH influence health, health behaviors, and health outcomes but also social interactions, quality of life, and life expectancy; and addressing SDOH can contribute to value-based health care delivery.[11,12]

There are multiple frameworks describing SDOH inclusive of factors such as marital status, income, educational level, employment and job insecurity, job opportunities, food insecurity, access to healthy foods, stable housing, neighborhood characteristics, built environment, physical activity opportunities, polluted air and water, transportation, childhood development, incarceration, and access to affordable health services.[5,6,11] *Healthy People 2030* categorize these social determinants into 5 domains:

- Economic stability
- Education access and quality
- Health care access and quality
- Neighborhood and built environment
- Social and community context

We characterize unique aspects of military service that impact the life course of veterans as they age, and how the military experience may alter health equity and health outcomes. Using the *Healthy People 2030* framework of SDOH, and the life-span model of the effects of military service and sociocultural dynamics and long-term outcomes of military service previously developed by Spiro,[13] **Fig. 1** contextualizes the trajectory of military service, SDOH, and access and use of VA and community resources and services to influence health equity and outcomes among older veterans. The outcomes include functionality in aging, morbidity, mortality, quality of life, and health care expenditures.

SOCIAL DETERMINANTS OF HEALTH IN RELATION TO VETERANS

Who are Our Veterans?

Veterans are former members of the Armed Forces of the United States which includes, Air Force, Navy, Marine Corps, Army, Coast Guard, and quite recently was expanded to include the National Guard. These individuals must have served on active

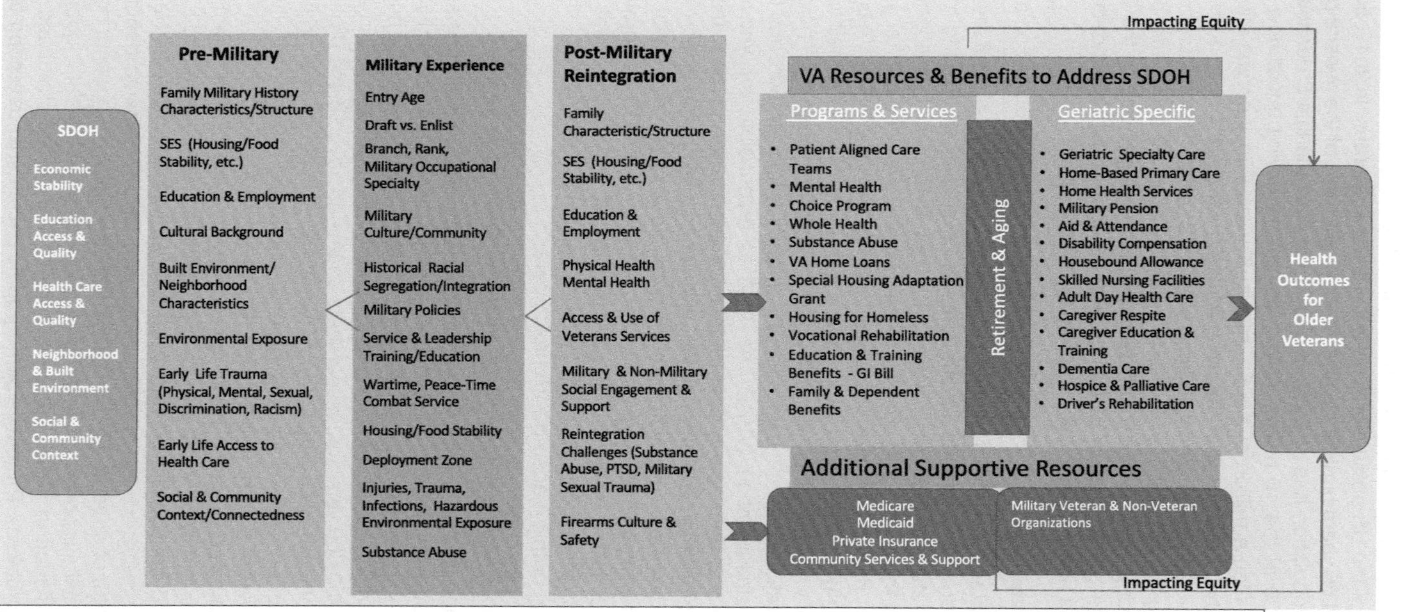

Fig. 1. SDOH & older veteran conceptual model. (*Adapted from*: Spiro et al, 2016 Long-term Outcomes of Military Service in aging and the life course: A positive re-envisioning.*Gerontologist*, 2016, Vol. 56, No. 1, 5–13.)

duty and were honorably discharged. Currently, there are approximately 18 million living US veterans, accounting for about 7% of the US population.[14] In comparison, in 1980, 38% of the US population over age 18 were veterans. In 2017, 54% of veterans were aged 65 years or older compared with only 18% of the general population.[15] The veteran population has changed significantly over the last 2 decades, with only around 240,000 of the 16 million WWII Veterans still living, most now in their late 90s, and less than a million of the 5.7 million Korean War Veterans alive according to data from the Department of Veterans Affairs.[16] Of the 8.7 million veterans of the Vietnam war, around 5.9 million are living. Members of this "baby boomer" generation started turning 65 in 2011, and in 2021, veterans aged 70 to 74 accounted for the largest age group of veterans. These demographic changes both in the veteran population and the US population overall create an urgent need for understanding and addressing the health challenges of an aging population.[17]

Services for Veterans

The United States Department of Veterans Affairs (VA) is an agency of the federal government that provides benefits, health care, and cemetery services to military veterans. The Secretary of Veterans Affairs, a cabinet-level official, is appointed by the President with the advice and consent of the Senate. VA is the federal government's second largest department after the Department of Defense.[18] The VA is responsible for administering benefit programs for veterans, their families, and their survivors. The Department of Veterans Affairs is made up of 3 main administrations: (1) Veterans Benefits Administration (VBA), (2) the National Cemetery Administration, and (3) the Veterans Health Administration (VHA). The VBA is responsible for veteran eligibility determination and VA's nonmedical benefits, which include home loans, insurance, vocational rehabilitation and employment, education and compensation and pension. The National Cemetery Administration manages veteran burial benefits. The VHA is one of the most expansive integrated health systems in the US and provides care to greater than 9 million veterans.[19] Less than half of all veterans seek care in the VHA, with much of their care received in the civilian health care system, and many veterans receiving both VA and non-VA health care.[15]

Disparities and Social Determinants of Health in Relation to Veterans

Evidence suggests that demographic disparities among nonveterans are the same factors that affect veterans. Patients from racial and ethnic minority groups are more likely to experience adverse SDOH such as housing instability, homelessness, food insecurity, and history of incarceration than White patients.[20–22] In a large study of more than 290,000 veterans, researchers examined adverse and protective SDOH and demographic characteristics among veterans. Their findings suggest that veterans from racial and ethnic minority groups, unmarried, and those with a service-connected disability were more likely to have cumulative adverse SDOH in 7 categories examined (violence, housing instability, employment or financial problems, legal problems, family or social support problems, access to care and transportation limitations, and nonspecific psychosocial needs). Veterans identified as non-White had 1.7 times greater odds of at least one adverse SDOH. Hispanic identified veterans had higher odds of adverse SDOH associated with violence, housing instability, and family and social support problems. Female veterans have greater odds of violence and family and support issues but lower odds of housing instability and employment and financial problems. Protective demographic characteristics among older age veterans were those that were married and residing in rural areas. Considering rurality, veterans residing in rural areas had a decreased likelihood of housing instability, employment/financial problems, family/social support problems, legal problems, and access to care and transportation.[23] These differences may exist as veterans living in rural areas tend to be older, married, experience less poverty, and have greater use of VA health care.[24]

When examining contextual factors affecting health that extend beyond health systems, SDOH change over one's lifespan. For example, childhood adversity and educational attainment are thought to influence military selection and military experience. When comparing men enlisting in the military during more recent eras compared with draft eras, there were higher rates of childhood adversity among veterans than nonveterans during nondraft eras.[1] Neighborhood determinants were also found to be important social factors among veterans receiving care at VHA that contribute to health disparities.[25] In a study looking at the impact of SDOH on hospitalization in VHA, researchers found among 360,527 veterans receiving care in primary care clinics, those living in neighborhoods with higher SES experience lower risk of hospitalization compared with veterans living in the lowest SES neighborhoods. Veterans hospitalized tended to be a mean age of 64.5 years.[9,10] Similarly, other researchers have found that individuals residing in impoverished neighborhoods had higher risk of hospital readmission.[26] This evidence provides support for the significant influence of SES on health outcomes and patterns of hospitalizations.

While military service and access to VA health care may be seen in some ways to "level the playing field" for those from disadvantaged backgrounds, some veterans may still experience inequity in achieving optimal health related to social determinants such as race or ethnicity, gender, sexual orientation, geographic location, socioeconomic status, mental health diagnoses, and disability. Research within VA has shown that racial and ethnic disparities in clinical outcomes and rates of chronic disease among veterans persist even when access and quality of care are comparable.[27] Black and Hispanic veterans, compared with White veterans, were more likely to depend on the VA to provide all or some of their care.[28] In a study comparing mortality of veterans who receive care in the VHA compared with the general population, disparities were noted for American Indian and Alaskan Native male VHA users not seen in the general US population.[21] Non-Hispanic Black men experience disparities in VHA and the general US population, though disparities were smaller in the VHA population. Non-Hispanic Black women users of VHA care had improved mortality compared with the general US population. Use of VA health care (vs VA nonuse) reduced, but did not eliminate, racial/ethnic disparities.[28]

Among the general population, racial and ethnic minority groups experience multiple barriers in accessing health care services and establishing usual sources of primary care. Veterans who use VHA services, including those from marginalized groups, have access to interdisciplinary team-based patient-centered primary care homes inclusive of social work, pharmacy, comprehensive mental health, and ancillary services such as physical and occupational therapy, and dietetics. Services such as transportation to VHA facilities, access to extended clinical hours, video telehealth and home care options, and onsite programs for legal, job rehabilitation, and housing support increased access for vulnerable veteran populations.[2–21] Accessing and using these VHA services are thought to reduce and attenuate health disparities among veterans from racial and ethnically diverse populations.[21] Given its mission, VHA recognized the need for additional resources to ensure equitable care to vulnerable populations with the creation of the VA Office of Health Equity, established in 2012, which champions the elimination of health disparities and achieving health equity for all veterans.[28]

OLDER VETERANS: A VULNERABLE POPULATION

Older veterans differ from the general US population and younger veteran cohorts in that they are less diverse, with 82% white (vs 62% for the non-Veteran population) and 97% male (vs 83% male for post-9/11 veterans).[16] The prevalence of certain health behaviors that are linked to chronic health conditions, such as smoking and obesity, is higher among veterans compared with nonveterans.[29] The prevalence of multiple chronic health conditions is higher than the general population for male (66.9% vs 61.9%) and female (74.1% vs 61.8%) veterans aged 65 and older.[29] While many older adults experience age-associated sensory, cognitive and physical declines, older veterans face an increased risk of chronic disease, geriatric syndromes such as falls, poly-pharmacy and cognitive impairment, and functional declines, some of which may emerge at earlier ages than in nonveteran patient populations.[17,30] Veterans are more likely to live with a functional disability (29% vs 13% nonveteran population), with 66% of disabled veterans aged 65 and older.[17] Care for older veterans requires attention not only to the challenges of aging, but also to the unique experiences and exposures of veterans that compound SDOH and manifest as HRSN which contribute to health outcomes in aging.

Older veterans may have unique experiences and exposures that affect their social, emotional, and physical health and how they age (**Table 1**). The effects of military service vary by era and conflict, with those serving in more recent eras experiencing greater adverse effects. Service in the military is often associated with negative effects such as physical injury, posttraumatic stress disorder (PTSD), substance abuse, and homelessness. In terms of mental health conditions, veterans who are enrolled in VHA care have overall higher rates of PTSD, alcohol use disorder, drug use disorder, and schizophrenia and lower rates of major depressive disorder and bipolar disorder, compared with the general US population.[15] Patients age 65 years and older enrolled in VHA care were less likely to have any mental health/substance use disorder outpatient visits (13.4%) compared with younger patients (32.4% for patients age 45-64 and 42.7% among patients age 18–44).[17] An estimated 5%-25% of veterans develop PTSD, with prevalence in younger veterans higher than that of older veterans.[31] The suicide rate among veterans was estimated to be 52% higher than the general US population in 2019, with veterans ages 55 to 74 the largest subgroup, accounting for 38% of veteran suicide deaths.[32] Importantly, military service can also positively affect a person's life trajectory. For example, the GI Bill allowed many veterans to achieve higher education and affordable housing, leading to higher SES.[13] Veterans, as a group, attain a higher level of education than the general population, and are more likely to have a high school or college degree. This holds true for minority veterans as well. Veterans are less likely to live in poverty, though minority veterans are more likely than nonminority veterans to live in poverty.[33]

Despite the positive effects of military service on subsequent education achievement, housing, employment, and SES of veterans relative to nonveterans and despite the constellation of services provided by VHA, many of which specifically target HRSN and care access, older veterans comprise a vulnerable patient population in which health inequities persist.[27] While metrics indicate VHA efforts to address HRSN are reducing disparities in mortality in veterans compared with nonveterans, racial/ethnic disparities among veterans using VHA exists.[34] Minority veteran men, for instance, were more likely to report combat exposure, a determinant that is associated with higher rates of several health conditions.[27]

We have (1) described SDOH and their potential protective or adverse influence on health and health outcomes; (2) characterized veterans in terms of SDOH and other

Table 1
Common military sevice-related health risks for older veterans

Ionizing Radiation Exposure/Nuclear Weapons	High risk for multiple cancers
Agent Orange Exposure	An herbicide used during the Vietnam era to destroy foliage. High risk for cancers (including respiratory and prostate cancer), type 2 diabetes, ischemic heart disease, soft tissue sarcoma, peripheral neuropathy
Camp Lejune Water Contamination	Tap water contaminated by industrial chemicals at Marine Corps Base Camp 1950s- 1980s. Increased risk for multiple cancers.
Hepatitis C	Exposures to blood and human fluids, group use of needles, razors, toothbrushes, and other personal items
Open Air Burns Pits	High risk for respiratory illnesses and wide variety of cancers, including leukemia
Noise Exposure	Hearing loss and tinnitus related to military noise exposures
Cold injuries	Extreme cold conditions leading to frost bite, neurologic or vascular injury
Traumatic brain injury	Caused by direct impact, rapid acceleration/ deceleration, or blast injuries sustained from traditional ordinance or improvised explosive device
Post-Traumatic Stress Disorder (PTSD)	May develop after experiencing or witnessing a life-threatening event
Military sexual trauma	Sexual assault or harassment experienced during military service
Depression and Suicide risk	Higher risk than the general population for men and women

Adapted from: https://www.publichealth.va.gov/PUBLICHEALTH/exposures/index.asp, https://www.va.gov/oaa/military-health-history-pocket-card.asp.

demographics; and (3) delineated the unique experiences, exposures, and consequent social and health vulnerabilities and inequities in veterans relative to the general population. Because SDOH and HRSN function to limit access to resources that otherwise protect and maintain individuals' health, it is not surprising that left unaddressed these social risk factors also limit the ability to reap the benefits of health interventions.[35,36] In this way care that fails to recognize and address SDOH and HRSN, which are key drivers of health inequities, can create new and compound existing disparities in patterns of health care utilization, morbidity, and mortality.

Greater understanding of the unique conditions and HRSN that can result from military service, in adjunct to SDOH, can support recognition and appropriately targeted treatment approaches.[37] Expanded understanding of the larger sociocultural contexts from which patients navigate their health self-management can not only support efforts to deliver patient-centered care but address, perhaps even eliminate, those barriers that may otherwise limit patients' ability to benefit optimally from that care. Practice-based opportunities for recognizing and addressing social needs in health care settings support patient-centered clinical decision making and care delivery[4–10]

Table 2
Key Recommendations and Tools to Identify and Address Social Determinants of Health in Older Veterans

Key Recommendations for Clinical Practice	Tool
1. Raise your awareness of who veterans are. →Familiarize yourself with the military specific exposures and health issues	*Refer to* ***Table 1*** Military Culture Core Competencies Course Review Profile of Veterans Report
2. Start the conversation: a. Evaluate Military Health History →Ask permission: "Would it be ok if I asked you about your military experience?" →Use the Military Health History Pocket Card questions to capture military experience and exposures b. Identify core patient goals and needs →Ask: "What matters most to you?"	Military Health History Pocket Card for Health Professions Trainees & Clinicians. https://www.va.gov/oaa/pocketcard/ Institute for Healthcare Improvement (2020). Age Friendly Health Systems: Guide to Using the 4Ms in the Care of Older Adults.
3. Identify unmet social needs →Employ a SDOH / HRSN Screening Tool	Selected SDOH Screening Tools are listed below
4. Address SDOH and /or unmet HRSN a. Provide veteran-specific information and resources for unmet social needs →Use items provided in **Table 3** b. Refer to appropriate social care services →VA Resources (**Table 3**) →Community Resources	*Resources for Veterans in* ***Table 3*** Veteran Community Partnerships National Resource Directory Neighborhood Navigator
5. Advocacy →Begin Conversation with Policy Stakeholders	Robert Wood Johnson Foundation: A New Way to Talk About the Social Determinants of Health: A New Way to Talk About the Social Determinants of Health

Selected SDOH Screening Tools

Name and Source	URL
PRAPARE Assessment Tool National Association of Community Health Centers	https://www.nachc.org/research-and-data/prapare/about-the-prapare-assessment-tool/
The Accountable Health Communities Screening Tool Center for Medicare & Medicaid Services	https://innovation.cms.gov/files/worksheets/ahcm-screeningtool.pdf
SDOH Tools & Resources Centers for Disease Control & Prevention	https://www.cdc.gov/socialdeterminants/tools/index.htm
Social Needs Screening Tool American Academy of Family Physicians	https://www.aafp.org/dam/AAFP/documents/patient_care/everyone_project/hops19-physician-form-sdoh.pdf

and may even have far reaching positive effects on age-related functional limitations.[38] Awareness of the benefits, services, and resources available for veterans and their caregivers (**Tables 2** and **3**) can support the efforts of providers and health professionals who care for them to provide patient centered, integrated care to optimally addresses the HRSN of older veterans.

Table 3
Selected resources to support older veterans and their families

VA Benefits and Eligibility Resources	
Information for Veterans	**Clinician note**
U.S. Department of Veterans Affairs: Veterans Benefits Administration https://benefits.va.gov 1- 800-698-2411	Eligibility for Veterans Administration benefits and programs
U.S. Department of Veterans Affairs: Veterans Health Administration (VHA) https://www.va.gov/health/ Health Benefits Hotline 1-877-222-8387	Health Benefits Information and Hotline
VHA Services for Aging Veterans VA Non-Medical Benefits for Older Veterans https://benefits.va.gov/PERSONA/ VA Health Care for Older Veterans https://www.va.gov/GERIATRICS/ Overview of VA Benefits for Older Veterans https://www.va.gov/files/2021-11/aging-veterans-quick-startguide.Pdf	
Specific Health Related Social Needs (HRSN) Support Resources	
Information for Veterans	*Clinician Tools /Information/Resources*
Now you just dial 988 then press 1 or Text 838255 TTY: https://www.veteranscrisisline.net/	If a Veteran is having thoughts of hurting themselves or ending their life get help right away. They, you, or a significant other can call the Crisis Line.
Food Insecurity https://www.nutrition.va.gov/Food_Insecurity.asp https://www.fns.usda.gov/military-and-veteran-families	Includes handouts for thrifty meals and nutrition tips for veterans without a home
VA Homeless Programs https://www.va.gov/HOMELESS/index.asp Call National Call Center for Homeless Veterans 1-877-424-3838 Brochure: https://www.va.gov/HOMELESS/docs/VA_Homeless_Brochure_AtRisk.pdf *Housing Assistance* https://www.va.gov/housing-assistance/	Comprehensive, individualized care to promote housing stability among Veterans who are homeless or at risk of becoming homeless. https://www.va.gov/HOMELESS/hchv.asp Outreach Tools: https://www.va.gov/HOMELESS/get_involved.asp
Employment *Veteran Readiness and Employment (VR&E)* https://www.benefits.va.gov/vocrehab/ *VA for Vets Veteran Employment Office* https://www.vaforvets.va.gov/	Support employment stability Formerly Vocational Rehabilitation and Employment
Military Sexual Trauma https://www.mentalhealth.va.gov/msthome/index.asp *Intimate Partner Violence Assistance Program* https://www.socialwork.va.gov/IPV/VETERANS_PARTNERS/Index.asp	Military Sexual Trauma education and outreach resources for community providers https://www.mentalhealth.va.gov/msthome/community-providers.asp
VA Mental Health Conditions, Symptoms, Substance Disorders,	Coaching into Care Program- Free service to assist with encouraging a Veteran to get

(*continued on next page*)

Table 3
(continued)

VA Benefits and Eligibility Resources	
Information for Veterans	**Clinician note**
Life Events https://www.maketheconnection.net/veterans/	support. Resources, referral, guidance -1-888-823-7458
PTSD – Post Traumatic Stress Disorder http://www.ptsd.va.gov	Information and resources
Women Veterans https://www.benefits.va.gov/PERSONA/veteran-women.asp https://www.va.gov/womenvet/	Information and resources
LGBTQ+ Veterans https://www.patientcare.va.gov/LGBT/index.asp	Information and resources
Minority Veterans https://www.benefits.va.gov/PERSONA/veteran-minority.asp	Resources, Programs and Benefits for African Americans, Asian American/Pacific Islander, Hispanic, Native American/Alaska Native and Native Hawaiian veterans.
Military Veteran Organizations & Legions https://militaryconnection.com/veterans/org/	Support Veterans to leverage social capitol and social support
VA Caregiver Support Services Caregiver Support Line at 855-260-3274 www.caregiver.va.gov	Information resources

ADDRESSING SOCIAL DETERMINANTS OF HEALTH

In order for health care providers to improve the health and health equity of vulnerable populations, such as older veterans, taking steps to identify and address SDOH and other HRSN is paramount. Two conceptual frameworks, in particular, may be helpful in thinking about how we can begin to address the adverse effects of SDOH and resulting inequities. The National Academies of Sciences, Engineering, and Medicine (NASEM) defined a framework with 5 activities or strategies that can be used by clinicians and systems to identify and address social risk factors.[39] These health care system activities include:

(1) Awareness – increase care team recognition of health-related social risk factors
(2) Adjustments – accommodate clinical decision-making social risk information
(3) Assistance – link patients with resources
(4) Alignment – facilitate synergy between health and social services
(5) Advocacy –engage health care sector in improvement efforts

Gurewich and colleagues[40] developed a conceptual framework, *Outcomes from Addressing SDoH in Systems (OASIS)*, to guide thinking about how the identification of and addressing unmet social needs can work to improve outcomes at several stages along a continuum. Specifically, unmet social needs can be identified by screening and referral for services to address unmet needs with possible direct and/or indirect positive impacts on outcomes. However, barriers to SDOH screening and intervention at the level of the patient, clinician, and health system have been identified.[41] These challenges include a concern regarding patient stigma and privacy, clinician lack of referral resources, and health system resource limitations for data collection and management. Likewise, commonly noted clinician concerns about addressing SDOH include limited time, insufficient skill for identifying social risks, and lack of referral networks for addressing identified determinants. A recent survey of 232 VHA Nurse practitioners, physicians, and physician assistants across 3 VA facilities identified "poor communication by providers" as a primary contributor to health care inequality (48%) and identified "time" and "resources" (60%) as organizational barriers for addressing social needs. Indeed, to successfully ameliorate SDOH driven health care disparities providers *and* systems must commit to addressing SDOH.[42] While the complexity of SDOH and the multiple levels of their influence[12] may make taking steps to address social needs daunting, adopting even small, micro-practice level changes in daily practice (see **Table 2**) can wield significant impacts in addressing SDOH and reducing health inequities.

Accruing evidence supports the contention that even *identifying* unmet social needs alone can support care. For instance, Zulman and colleagues[43] augmented electronic health record data with patient-reported SDOH; an approach that consistently improved 90-day and 180-day hospital admission risk estimation in a sample of high-risk veterans. Others have demonstrated that the integration of HRSN services, supports and community partnerships reduce emergency department use by veterans receiving homeless services by 19% at 6-month follow-up with a reduction of 34.7% in hospitalization.[44]

Approaches to Identify Unmet Social Determinants of Health and Health-Related Social Needs

There is limited evidence-based guidance for how to best screen for SDOH/HRSN, despite the availability of a multitude of screening tools.[41] However, some practical recommendations for identifying SDOH/HRSN with older veterans follow and a listing of selected multidimensional screening tools is provided in **Table 2**.

Starting the conversation

While the following "conversation starters" are not formalized as SDOH screening items, we recommend using this set of key questions to identify military-related social risks and exposures that may exert adverse effects on health. These Military Health History questions should be used with older veterans even if a formalized SDOH/HRSN screening tool is used in adjunct to support timely referral to specialized services if needed. The following items are abstracted from the VHA Office of Academic Affiliations' *Military Health History Pocket Card for Health Professions Trainees and Clinicians* available at https://www.va.gov/OAA/archive/Military-Health-History-Card-for-print.pdf [45]

Explain: I have some questions that will help me understand your health history.
Ask:

- *Did you serve in the Military? Which branch? What was your job?*
- *Would it be ok to ask you about your military service?*
- *During your military service, were you exposed to noise, chemicals, or other hazardous substances?*
- *Did you have any unwanted sexual experiences during your military service?*
- *Do you receive any benefits from VA?*
- *Would it be ok to ask about your living situation?*
    - *Do you have a safe place to go to when you leave today?*
- *Have you had thoughts of harming yourself?*

In settings whereby the opportunity for the administration of a formalized SDOH screening is extremely limited, a cursory approach may be to ask patients the Institute for Healthcare Improvement Age Friendly Health System 4 Ms[46] question *"What matters most to you?".* Intended to be used as a set, the IHI 4 Ms questions work to identify core issues to support the care of older adults. "What Matters" enables the alignment of care with patient care goals and preferences, and assuming that individuals have a propensity for identifying basic order needs (eg, food insecurity, housing instability) before higher order needs[40] (eg, medication refills), may well elicit conversation regarding unmet HRSN. While studies are needed, vulnerable populations bearing significant adverse HRSN burden may disclose food insecurity, housing, and safety concerns to trigger social work and other interdisciplinary consults and referral.

Screening

Available SDOH/HRSN screening tools are plentiful and capture an array of social risk factors and needs. A recent technical brief for the US Preventive Services Task Force addressed screening and interventions for social risk factors and noted wide variation among the many multidomain social risk screening tools that have been developed.[41,47,48] Most of these are self-report formats and most have not been validated. The VHA Office of Health Equity supported the development of ACORN (Assessing Circumstances and Offering Resources for Needs), an 11-item screening assessment that is part of a quality improvement initiative to screen veterans for nonclinical social needs that may be impacting their health.[49] ACORN screens for 9 domains including food, housing, utility, and transportation insecurities; educational, employment and legal needs; personal safety; loneliness and social isolation; and lack of phone/Internet or technology access (digital divide). See **Table 2** for additional screening resources.

Addressing Unmet Social Determinants of Health and Health-Related Social Needs

Once unmet SDOH/HRSN are identified referral to social care services and specific resources targeting identified unmet social needs should naturally follow. Awareness of the benefits, services, and resources available for veterans and their caregivers, in VHA and the greater community, can support the efforts of health professionals who care for older veterans to provide comprehensive patient-centered care that integrates strategies for addressing unmet HRSN in the care plan.

Specific approaches include developing resource guides that can be provided to patients and families. The National Resource Directory (www.nrd.gov), for instance is a vetted searchable online collection of national and local programs, services, and organizations for veterans and their families organized by categories including benefits and compensation, transportation, homeless assistance, disability services, legal and financial assistance, women's resources, veteran service organizations, military sexual trauma, and more. The Neighborhood Navigator EveryONE Project website (https://www.aafp.org/family-physician/patient-care/the-everyone-project/neighborhood-navigator.html), developed by the American Academy of Family Physicians, is an interactive, online tool that can be used at the point of care to help clinicians address unmet social needs by identifying and connecting patients to needed social services in their area including food, transportation, housing, legal aid, employment aid, and financial assistance. See **Tables 2** and **3** for additional resources for health professionals and for veterans and their families, respectively.

PARTNERING TO ADDRESS SOCIAL DETERMINANTS OF HEALTH/HEALTH-RELATED SOCIAL NEEDS: SOCIAL WORK

It has been suggested that "the levels of health inequity that currently exist in the US will not be relieved by one health care profession alone".[50] Interprofessional collaboration is fundamental to health care delivery that accomplishes social needs care integration effectively. However, most medical and health professions curricula have not traditionally integrated SDOH, and when present competencies in SDOH are not taught in ways that foster interprofessional collaborative practice despite established interprofessional education and training paradigms. A recent study[51] with 768 nurses reported that knowledge and confidence for integrating SDOH in everyday practice were limited by unfamiliarity with resources for referral. Study participants expressed the need for interdisciplinary collaboration and information regarding the role of social workers. The integration of social workers as part of interprofessional primary care teams was demonstrated to improve the feasibility of assessment, management and reevaluation of vulnerable patients' HRSN and improved overall care team effectiveness. In fact, when social workers were added to VHA rural primary care teams a 3% reduction in emergency department visits and 4.4% decrease in acute hospital admissions were seen[52] as well as reductions in care fragmentation and adverse outcomes in patients using both VHA and community-based care.[53] (O'Brien, 2019) discusses the vital role of social work in addressing SDOH.[47] Social workers are trained to address social and economic disparities across the continuum of care, including identifying appropriate community-based interventions, connecting patients with resources and services, and conducting a subsequent evaluation for outcomes and follow-up as well as training care teams in protocols for screening, intervention, and referral.

NURSES POSITIONALITY FOR ADVOCACY: FOSTERING HEALTH EQUITY

The SDOH are a set of intersecting complex factors on an individual and community/population level which require advocacy and leadership to prompt culture and policy change across multiple sectors (local, state, and federal agencies, academia) and in partnership with stakeholders and interdisciplinary colleagues[3–30,31–54] to improve health equity. Nurses at all levels are uniquely poised to lead efforts to address SDOH, health inequities and disparities, and social injustices including discriminatory practices and racism within practice, research, education, and policies across health systems and institutions to advance health equity among patients, families, and communities.[54,55]

SUMMARY

Achieving health equity among older veterans requires interdisciplinary teams to identify and address complex social issues that contribute to health disparities. The influence of SDOH and military service are interconnected and considered together provide important opportunities to support veterans' aging, health and health outcomes. Focusing on medical care interventions only does not address the breadth of patient care needs to advance health equity among vulnerable populations. Nurses are central to interdisciplinary team approaches to address SDOH across all health care settings and advocate for structural and policy changes that improve health outcomes for all older adults.

CLINICS CARE POINTS

- Health care providers should ask about and document patient's military service status and complete a military service history if they have served.

- Nurses are integral to interdisciplinary team approaches to assessing and addressing SDOH to advance health equity.
- Screening tools are available to identify unmet social needs in the clinical setting.
- To effectively address HRSN of older veterans, health care providers should be familiar with VA benefits and VA/community resources.

ACKNOWLEDGMENTS

Sincere gratitude to Robert Jones III, Command Sergeant Major, Retired for his personal contribution to this article.

DISCLOSURE

All authors have no commercial or financial conflicts to disclose.

The contents of this article do not represent the views of Department of Veterans Affairs or the US government.

REFERENCES

1. Duan-Porter W, Martinson BC, Taylor B, et al. Evidence review: social determinants of health for veterans. J Gen Intern Med 2018;33(10):1785–95.
2. Blosnich JR, Dichter ME, Gurewich D, et al. Health services research and social determinants of health in the nation's largest integrated health care system: steps and leaps in the veterans health administration. Mil Med 2020;185(9–10):e1353–6.
3. Center for Disease Control and Prevention. NCHHSTP social determinants of health. 2019. Available at: https://www.cdc.gov/nchhstp/socialdeterminants/index.html.
4. Center for Disease Control and Prevention. Social determinants of health and alzheimers disease and related dementias. 2020. Available at: https://www.cdc.gov/aging/disparities/social-determinants-alzheimers.html.
5. Center for Disease Control and Prevention. Social determinants of health. 2021. Available at: https://www.cdc.gov/chronicdisease/programs-impact/sdoh.htm.
6. World Health Organization (n.d. Social determinants of health. Available at: https://www.who.int/health-topics/social-determinants-of-health#tab=tab_1.
7. Cantor MN, Thorpe L. Integrating data on social determinants of health into electronic health records. Health Aff 2018;37(4):585–90. https://doi.org/10.1377/hlthaff.2017.1252.
8. Davis CI, Montgomery AE, Dichter ME, et al. Social determinants and emergency department utilization: findings from the veterans health administration. Am J Emerg Med 2020;38(9):1904–9.
9. Hatef E, Searle KM, Predmore Z, et al. The impact of social determinants of health on hospitalization in the veterans health administration. Am J Prev Med 2019;56(6):811–8. https://doi.org/10.1016/j.amepre.2018.12.012.
10. Hatef E, Predmore Z, Lasser EC, et al. Integrating social and behavioral determinants of health into patient care and population health at Veterans Health Administration: a conceptual framework and an assessment of available individual and population level data sources and evidence-based measurements. AIMS public health 2019;6(3):209–24. https://doi.org/10.3934/publichealth.2019.3.209.

11. U.S. Department of Health and Human Services (N.D. A). Healthy people 2030. Available at: https://health.gov/healthypeople/about/workgroups/social-determinants-health-workgroup.
12. Johnson Foundation Robert Wood. A new way to talk about the social determinants of health. 2010. Available at: https://www.rwjf.org/en/library/research/2010/01/a-new-way-to-talk-about-the-social-determinants-of-health.html.
13. Spiro Settersten, Aldwin. Long-term outcomes of military service in aging and the life course: a positive re-envisioning. Gerontologist 2016;56(1):5–13.
14. Vespa Jonathan E. Those who served: America's veterans from World war II to the war on terror," ACS-43. Washington, DC: American Community Survey Reports, U.S. Census Bureau; 2020.
15. National healthcare quality and disparities report chartbook on healthcare for veterans. Rockville, MD: Agency for Healthcare Research and Quality; 2020. AHRQ Pub. No. 21-000.
16. National center for veterans analysis and statistics (va.gov. Available at: https://www.va.gov/vetdata/report.asp. Accessed December 21, 2021.
17. VA Office of Health Equity. National veteran health equity report—FY2013. Washington, DC: US Department of Veterans Affairs; 2016. Available online at. http://www.va.gov/healthequity/NVHER.asp.
18. Office of Rural Health. About us. (n.d.) Available at: https://www.ruralhealth.va.gov/aboutus/structure.asp Accessed 12/21/21
19. Veterans Health Administration. (n.d.) Available at: https://www.va.gov/health/Accessed 12/21/21
20. Montgomery AE, Szymkowiak D, Tsai J. Housing instability and homeless program use among veterans: the intersection of race, sex, and homelessness. Housing Policy Debate 2020;30(3):396–408.
21. Wong MS, Hoggatt KJ, Steers WN, et al. Racial/ethnic disparities in mortality across the Veterans health administration. Health Equity 2019;3(1):99–108.
22. Steiner JF, Stenmark SH, Sterrett AT, et al. Food insecurity in older adults in an integrated health care system. J Am Geriatr Soc 2018;66(5):1017–24.
23. Montgomery AE, Tsai J, Blosnich JR. Demographic correlates of veterans' adverse social determinants of health. Am J Prev Med 2020;59(6):828–36.
24. Holder KA. Veterans in rural America: 2011–2015. Washington, DC: US Department of Commerce, Economics and Statistics Administration, US Census Bureau; 2017.
25. Wong MS, Steers WN, Hoggatt KJ, et al. Relationship of neighborhood social determinants of health on racial/ethnic mortality disparities in US veterans-Mediation and moderating effects. Health Serv Res 2020;55(Suppl 2):851–62. https://doi.org/10.1111/1475-6773.13547.
26. Hu J, Gonsahn MD, Nerenz DR. Socioeconomic status and readmissions: evidence from an urban teaching hospital. Health Aff 2014;33(5):778–85.
27. Ward RE, Nguyen X-MT, Li Y, et al. Racial and ethnic disparities in U.S. veteran health characteristics. Int J Environ Res Public Health 2021;18:2411. https://doi.org/10.3390/ijerph18052411.
28. VA Office of Health Equity. VHA office of health equity. 2020. Available at: https://www.va.gov/healthequity/.
29. Boersma P, Cohen RA, Zelaya CE, et al. Multiple chronic conditions among veterans and nonveterans: United States, 2015–2018. national health statistics reports. Hyattsville, MD: National Center for Health Statistics; 2021. https://doi.org/10.15620/cdc:101659. no 153.

30. Howard JT, Janak JC, Santos-Lozada AR, et al. Telomere shortening and accelerated aging in US Military veterans. Int J Environ Res Public Health 2021;18: 1743. https://doi.org/10.3390/ijerph18041743.
31. Institute of Medicine. Returning home from Iraq and Afghanistan: assessment of readjustment needs of veterans, service members, and their families. Washington, DC: The National Academies Press; 2013.
32. Office of Mental Health and Suicide Prevention. National veterans suicide prevention annual report. 2021. Available at: https://www.mentalhealth.va.gov/docs/data-sheets/2021/2021-National-Veteran-Suicide-Prevention-Annual-Report-FINAL-9-8-21.pdf.
33. Minority veterans report: military service history and va benefit utilization statistics. data governance and analytics. Washington, DC: Department of Veterans Affairs; 2017.
34. Office of Health Equity Veterans Health Administration Department of Veterans Affairs. Identifying and addressing health related social needs among veterans fact sheets. Available at: https://www.va.gov/HEALTHEQUITY/docs/Social_Determinants_Fact_Sheet_V2-0.pdf.
35. Resnicow K, Braithwaite RL, Dilorio C, et al. Applying theory to culturally diverse and unique populations. In: Glanz K, Lewis FM, Rimer BK, editors. Health behavior and health education: theory, research, and practice. 3rd Edition. San Francisco: Jossey-Bass Publishers; 2002. p. 485–509.
36. Alcántara C, Diaz SV, Cosenzo LG, et al. Social determinants as moderators of the effectiveness of health behavior change interventions: scientific gaps and opportunities. Health Psychol Rev 2020;14(1):132–44. https://doi.org/10.1080/17437199.2020.1718527.
37. Richard-Eaglin A, Campbell JG, Utley-Smith Q. The aging veteran population: promoting awareness to influence best practices. Geriatr Nurs 2020;41:505507. https://doi.org/10.1016/j.gerinurse.
38. Rhee TG, Marottoli RA, Cooney LM Jr, et al. Associations of social and behavioral determinants of health index with self-rated health, functional limitations, and health services use in older adults. J Am Geriatr Soc 2020;68:1731–8. https://doi.org/10.1111/jgs.16429.
39. Razon NA, Hessler D, Bibbins-Domingo K, et al. How hypertension guidelines address social determinants of health: a systematic scoping review. Med Care 2021;59(12):1122–9.
40. Gurewich D, Garg A, Kressin NR. Addressing social determinants of health within healthcare delivery systems: a framework to ground and inform health outcomes. J Gen Intern Med 2020;35(5):1571.
41. Eder M, Henninger M, Durbin S, et al. Screening and interventions for social risk factors: technical brief to support the US preventive services task force. JAMA 2021;326(14):1416–28.
42. Partin MR, TaylorBrent C, Gordon HS, et al. Veterans affairs providers' beliefs about the contributors to and responsibility for reducing racial and ethnic health care disparities. Health equity 2019;3(1):436–48.
43. Zulman DM, Maciejowski ML, Grubber JM, et al. Patient-reported social and behavioral determinants of health and estimated risk of hospitalization in high-risk veterans affairs patients. JAMA Netw open 2020;3(10):e2021457.
44. O'Toole TP, Johnson EE, Aiello R, et al. Tailoring care to vulnerable populations by incorporating social determinants of health: the veterans health administration's "homeless patient aligned care team" program. Prev Chronic Dis 2016;13: 150567. https://doi.org/10.5888/pcd13.150567.

45. VHA Office of Academic Affiliations. Military health history pocket card for health professions trainees and clinicians. 2019. Available at: https://www.va.gov/OAA/archive/Military-Health-History-Card-for-print.pdf.
46. Institute for Healthcare Improvement. Age friendly health systems: guide to using the 4ms in the care of older adults. 2020. Available at: http://www.ihi.org/Engage/Initiatives/Age-Friendly-Health-Systems/Documents/IHIAgeFriendlyHealthSystems_GuidetoUsing4MsCare.pdf.
47. O'Brien KH. Social determinants of health: the how, who, and where screenings are occurring; a systematic review. Social Work Health Care 2019;58(8):719–45.
48. Elias RR, Jutte DP, Moore A. Exploring consensus across sectors for measuring the social determinants of health. SSM-population health 2019;7:100395.
49. Cohen AJ, Lehmann LS, Russell LE. Systematic screening of veterans for health-related social needs: an ethical imperative. Health Services Research & Development; 2020.
50. Thornton M, Persaud S. Preparing today's nurses: social determinants of health and nursing education. OJIN: Online J Issues Nurs 2018;23(No. 3). Manuscript 5.
51. Phillips J, Richard A, Mayer KM, et al. Integrating the social determinants of health into nursing practice: nurses' perspectives. J Nurs Scholarsh 2020; 52(5):497–505. https://doi.org/10.1111/jnu.12584. Epub 2020 Jul 11. PMID: 32654364.
52. Cornell, PY et al., (2020) doi: 10.1377/hlthaff.2019.01589. HEALTH AFFAIRS 39, NO. 4 (2020): 603–612. DOI: https://doi.org/10.21203/rs.3.rs-783581/v1
53. Sjoberg H, Lui W, Rohs C, et al. Optimizing care coordination to address social determinants of health needs for dual-use veterans. BMC Health Serv Res 2021;22(1):59.
54.. National Academies of Sciences, Engineering, and Medicine. The future of nursing 2020-2030, . Charting a Path to Achieve Health Equity. Washington, DC: The National Academies Press; 2021.
55. American Nurses Association. The national commission to address racism in nursing reflects on nurses' vast contributions during nurses month. 2021. Retrieved from. https://www.nursingworld.org/news/news-releases/2021/the-national-commission-to-address-racism-in-nursing-reflects-on–nurses-vast-contributions-during-nurses-month/.

Identifying Suicide Risk Factors in Lesbian, Gay, Bisexual, Transgender, and Queer Veterans

Sherley Belizaire, DNP, PMHNP-BC, FNP-BC[a,*],
Alexis Dickinson, PMHNP-BC[a], Michelle Webb, DNP, RN, BC-CHPCA[b]

KEYWORDS

• Veterans • LGBTQ • Suicide risk • Assessment • Intersectionality

KEY POINTS

- Lesbian, gay, bisexual, transgender, and queer (LGBTQ) veterans are at higher risk for suicide than the general population.
- The identification of suicide risk factors is the first step in developing a safety plan and recommended course of treatment that promotes healing and prevents further psychological and physiologic injury.
- It is critical for health care professionals to establish trusting relationships with LGBTQ veterans to better assess their suicide risk and mental health needs.
- Safety planning and coordination of care between the primary care, mental health, and VA provider, if there is one, are important strategies for reducing the risk of suicide in LGBTQ veterans.

BACKGROUND

Suicide is a major public health problem that affects people irrespective of age, race and ethnicity, gender, veteran status,[1,2,] or sexual orientation.[1] According to the Centers for Disease Control and Prevention, suicide rates are higher among sexual and gender minorities and veterans than the general population in the United States (US).[3] Lesbian and bisexual females are 2 times more likely to attempt suicide than their heterosexual female peers. It is even higher in gay and bisexual males, four times more than their heterosexual male peers.[4] Among the veteran population, transgender veterans were 2 times more likely to die of suicide than their cisgender veteran peers, and more than

[a] Nurse Practitioner Residency Program-Mental Health, U.S. Department of Veteran Affairs, VA Boston Healthcare System, 940 Belmont Street, Brockton, MA 02301, USA; [b] Duke University School of Nursing, 307 Trent Drive, Durham, NC 27710, USA
* Corresponding author.
E-mail address: sherley.belizaire@va.gov

Nurs Clin N Am 57 (2022) 347–358
https://doi.org/10.1016/j.cnur.2022.04.003
0029-6465/22/Published by Elsevier Inc.

five times that of the general population.[5] The US Department of Veterans Affairs (VA), 2021 National Veteran Suicide Prevention Annual Report found that in 2019 the adjusted suicide rate among veterans was 52.3% higher than the nonveteran population.[6] The greatest unadjusted suicide rates were in white veterans, male veterans, and veterans aged 18 to 34. Younger veterans aged 18 to 34 were 1.65 times more likely to die by suicide than any other age group in the veteran population. Among veterans who died from suicide, more than 50% of them were not seen within the VA.[6] The purpose of this article is to provide an overview of risk and protective factors for suicide in the lesbian (L), gay (G), bisexual (B), transgender (T), and queer (Q) veteran population, identify the tools and resources necessary to address their mental health needs, and outline an evidence-based approach for community health care professionals to use as a guide for treatment and suicide prevention in this unique population.

EPIDEMIOLOGY

Annually, more than 700,00 people die by suicide worldwide.[2] In 2019, suicide was the 10th leading cause of premature mortality for all ages in the US. It was the second and fourth leading cause of death among people aged 10 to 34 and 35 to 44, respectively, higher than deaths due to homicide. The fifth leading cause of death among people aged 45 to 54 was suicide.[7] Approximately, 12 million adults contemplated suicide, 3.5 million formulated a suicide plan, 1.4 million attempted suicide, and more than 47,000 died as a result of suicide.[1] Women were 1.66 times more likely to attempt suicide; however, men were 3.63 times more likely to die as a result of suicide.[8] It is plausible that more men died from suicide because the most common method used was more lethal. Among men of all ages, 55.6% of suicide deaths were due to firearms. Whereas the most common method used among women aged 15 to 24 (45.3%), 25 to 34 (38.4%), and 35 to 44 (33.3%) was suffocation. For women aged 45 to 54, poisoning was the most common method used, accounting for 34.8% of suicides.[7] The lesbian, gay, bisexual, transgender, and queer (LGBTQ) population is a group disproportionally affected by suicide and has a greater rate of suicide than their heterosexual peers.[3,9] Young LGB individuals aged 18 to 25 had a higher rate of suicide ideation (27.9%), suicide plan (11.5%), and suicide attempt (5.5%) than the adult LGB aged 26 to 49 suicide ideation (14.5%), suicide plan (5.7%), and suicide attempt (2.2%).[10] Regarding the veteran population, the suicide rate (31.6 per 100,000) was greater than the general adult population (16.8 per 100,000).[6] With respect to race and ethnicity, Caucasians (15.67%) and American Indian/Alaskan Native (13.64%) had a higher rate of suicide in comparison to Black or African Americans (7.04%) and Asians and Pacific Islanders (7.04%).[11]

SUICIDE RISK ASSESSMENT

The Role of Intersectionality in the Lesbian, Gay, Bisexual, Transgender, and Queer Veteran Experience/Suicide Risk

An important consideration in the comprehensive assessment of the unique care needs of LGBTQ veterans at risk for suicide is the role of intersectionality or "how one's intersecting identities affect the way one perceives the world and how one interacts with it."[12(p.113)] In 2 seminal essays in 1989 and 1991, Dr Kimberle Williams Crenshaw, a black feminist scholar, began to use the term "intersectionality" to address the overlapping nature of problems like racism and sexism and the multiple levels of social injustice they can create and perpetuate.[12,13] Introduced initially to the field of legal studies, Crenshaw's exploration and concept definition centered on the oppression of black women in society and the ways in which they experience discrimination at the intersection of their 2 distinct social identities. Today, the concept of intersectionality has been applied to analyze and understand the unique experiences of discrimination and oppression associated with numerous other social identities. Unique experiences of discrimination such as microaggressions, provider bias, inequitable care and treatment, and marginalization have been commonly ascribed to race and gender as well as other social identities including sexual orientation, class, ability, nationality, citizenship, religion, and body type. Intersectionality provides an analytical framework for understanding how these identities combine and contribute to individual experiences of discrimination and privilege that can impact overall mental health.

As the veteran population and the LGBTQ population become increasingly diverse, it is essential that each LGBTQ veteran be viewed as a complex individual existing in a variety of systems and holding many intersecting identities which contribute to multidimensionality of lived experience that may increase the risk of suicidal behavior. The lived experiences of the LGBTQ veteran population may reflect what has been described as a "process of dehumanization"[(p.114)] for those who do not fit the patriarchal dominant culture that exists in the active military and ultimately transfers to the broader veteran culture.[14] For example, women veterans experience negative health care outcomes, retraumatization, and marginalization during the community reintegration process and an increased prevalence of sexual trauma and posttraumatic stress syndrome compared with their male counterparts and nonveterans.[15–17]

Knowledge of existing disparities in health, health care, and social experiences for LGBTQ veterans is key to identifying the relevant psychological and social determinants of their mental health. Mental health providers widely acknowledge the significance of social determinants of mental health to the etiology and epidemiology of mental illness.[18,19] The increased prevalence of substance misuse, depression, and suicidal attempts/ideation among LGBTQ persons; the intersecting aspect of relationship dynamics and LGBTQ veteran status tend to exacerbate service-related trauma.[20] LGBTQ individuals experience intimate partner violence at higher rates than the general population[21] and health care inequities and provider bias are well-documented among LGBTQ and other historically marginalized groups.[21,22] Furthermore, identity intersectionality plays a role in suicide risk; the highest rate of suicide attempts within the LGBTQ community is among African American, Latino, Native American, and Asian American individuals.[4] Therefore, careful consideration of the impact and interplay of the intersecting identities of LGBTQ veterans is a required element of a comprehensive assessment of risk of self-harm and suicidal risk. Through the application of intersectionality theory, various aspects of a veteran's identity can be examined to ensure patient-centered, culturally, and trauma-informed assessment, care planning, and intervention are achieved.

Lesbian, Gay, Bisexual, Transgender, and Queer-Specific Risk and Protective Factors

In addition to risk factors, warning signs, and protective factors (**Table 1**)[23] for the general population, clinicians must consider factors specific to the LGBTQ population when assessing suicide risk. These unique risk factors include family rejection, prejudice and discrimination in daily life as well as in laws and policies, bullying, violence, and sexual abuse.[4] Additionally, coming out is a particularly risky time for LGBTQ individuals given that they often feel the most depressed before coming out, and family rejection postdisclosure can multiply suicide risk by 8.[4] LGBTQ individuals who have experienced family rejection and community discrimination often feel isolated and experience worsening mental health symptoms.[4] One study found that feelings of attempted but unsuccessful belongingness, or the perception that the individual is a burden, predicted increased levels of suicidal ideation.[5] However, several studies

Table 1
Suicide risk assessment

Risk Factors	Warning Signs	Protective Factors
• Presence of mental health and/or substance use disorders • Poor access to or stigma associated with mental health treatment • Feelings of hopelessness • Impulsive tendencies • Personal history of suicide attempt • Family history or exposure to others who have died by suicide • Recent loss of finances, job, or relationship • Social isolation • LGBTQ identity • History of trauma • Chronic illness • Access to lethal means	• Talking about feeling hopeless or trapped, or wanting to die • Feeling like a burden to others • Increased anxiety or agitation • Social withdrawal • Increased substance use or reckless behavior • Mood swings • Change in sleep • Planning or researching ways to kill oneself	• Access to effective treatment of all health problems • Connection to family, community, medical, and mental health supports • Problem-solving skills • Cultural and religious beliefs that instill hope and discourage suicide • Restricted access to lethal means

Data from Suicide Awareness Voices of Education. Warning Signs of Suicide. Available at https://save.org/about-suicide/warning-signs-risk-factors-protective-factors/. Accessed November 16, 2021.

have shown that psychosocial support groups connecting minority individuals have been found to reduce the negative consequences of rejection, discrimination, and minority violence.[4,5] Specifically within the veteran population, transgender veterans who are actively connected to the larger veteran community have been found to have lower levels of suicidal ideation.[4,24] Further, connection to social groups in which an individual experiences support, belonging, acceptance, while interacting with positive role models has been found to promote resilience. When a person feels group belonging, self-worth and hope begin to build, and mental health improves.[24] Additional protective factors specific to the LGBTQ population include family acceptance of identity, a sense of safety in the community, connections to people who are accepting and care about that person, access to LGBTQ-affirming mental health treatment and reduction in symptoms of mental health or substance use disorders.[4]

The LGBTQ community has higher documented rates of anxiety, depression, and mood disorders than the general population; however, differences in mental health diagnoses are not the result of an inherent difference in the LGBTQ population, but instead reflect the impact of consistent stigma, discrimination, and minority stress.[25–27] It has been well documented that members of minority groups experience external stressors such as rejection and discrimination that impact their mental health, well-being, and internal beliefs which can perpetuate internalized shame.[26] LGBTQ individuals who have experienced verbal or physical harassment are at more than twice the risk of harming themselves than their peers who have not experienced this type of harassment.[4]

LGBTQ veterans are exposed to even higher rates of trauma than both their non-LGBTQ veteran and nonveteran LGBTQ peers.[25] In addition to military-specific traumas such as exposure to violence and combat, military sexual trauma, and separation from loved ones, LGBTQ veterans are also exposed to victimization, isolation, feeling pressure to conceal their identity, and being harassed based on their sexual and/or gender identity.[25] This increased exposure to trauma has a direct impact on LGBTQ veteran's mental health, for example, transgender-related discrimination for individuals serving in the military has been found to be indirectly related to suicidal ideation and shame about identity.[5]

Despite the additional risk factors, trauma, and higher rates of anxiety and mood disorders seen within the LGBTQ population, this group has more difficulty accessing health care and is less likely to stay engaged with health care than their heterosexual counterparts related to fear of discrimination and current or previous experience with prejudice from providers.[28,29] Therefore, it is critical for health care professionals to establish trusting relationships with LGBTQ veterans to better assess their mental health and suicide risk.

CLINICAL ASSESSMENT OF SUICIDE RISK

General Guidelines

The Joint Commission released recommendations for suicide screening in 2016 to guide the assessment and screening of suicidality.[30] These recommendations included the utilization of 5 different evidenced-based suicide screening tools: the Patient Health Questionnaire-9 (PHQ-9), Patient Health Questionnaire-2 (PHQ-2), Suicide Behaviors Questionnaire-Revised (SBQ-R), Columbia-Suicide Severity Rating Scale (C-SSRS), and ED-SAFE Patient Safety Screener-3 (PSS-3).[30] The PHQ-9 screens for diagnosis and severity of depression, as well as the presence of suicidal ideation and has a high level of specificity. The PHQ-2 is an abbreviated version of the PHQ-9.[30] The SBQ-R has high sensitivity and specificity. It screens for the history of suicidal ideation and attempt, suicidal ideation over the past year, whether the individual told anyone that he or she had plans to end his or her life by suicide, and a self-reported likelihood that the individual will attempt suicide in the future.[30] The C-SSRS has been shown to predict suicidal behavior in adults and adolescents.[30] It assesses the severity of suicidal ideation, presence of suicidal behavior, and previous suicide attempts. The PSS-3 has been widely studied and includes a scripted introduction to be used with the patient before asking about depressed mood, suicidal ideation, and history of suicide attempts.[30]

Veterans Affairs Guidelines

As part of the National Strategy for Preventing Veteran Suicide 2018 to 2028, the VA implemented Suicide Risk Identification Strategy (Risk ID) a strategy to ensure all veterans accessing VA health care are screened for suicide at least annually as a part of a larger effort to prevent veteran suicide.[31] These guidelines state that all veterans must be screened at least annually for suicide risk in any clinic; however, veterans should also be screened for suicide whenever it is clinically indicated, including at every mental health appointment.[31] Risk ID breaks down suicide screening into 3 steps: first complete a PHQ-9. This can be conducted at least annually. If the veteran answers yes to number 9 on the PHQ-9 then complete a C-SSRS. Finally, if the veteran screens positive on the C-SSRS, complete a Comprehensive Suicide Risk Evaluation (CSRE).[31] The results of the CSRE will determine the next course of action and treatment plan. The CSRE is a more detailed assessment of suicide risk which involves asking about evidence-based factors including risk and protective factors, suicidal behaviors, ideation, plan, and intent which helps the health care provider to determine a veteran's acute and chronic risk for suicide and most appropriate level of care.[31]

RECOMMENDATIONS

When establishing a treatment plan for LGBTQ veterans with suicidal ideation, intent, and/or behavior, important considerations include determining the appropriate level of care, establishing a safety plan, and understanding the underlying diagnoses and stressors triggering suicidal thoughts.[32] LGBTQ veterans endorsing suicidal ideation with intent to die by suicide and cannot maintain safety in the community warrant inpatient hospitalization.[32] Health care professionals should work with veterans to maintain their safety in the community and develop a patient-centered and evidenced-based treatment plan.[32] This plan may include a combination of psychotherapy, psychopharmacology, and care coordination between primary care, mental health, and/or VA providers.[32]

The Education Corps of the VA Center of Excellence for Suicide Prevention developed the VA S.A.V.E. training that helps veterans and health care professionals who care for veterans recognize and identify veterans at risk for suicide.[33] The S.A.V.E acronym stands for S ("Signs of suicidal thinking should be recognized"), A ("Ask the most important question of all"—"Are you thinking of killing yourself?"), V ("Validate the Veteran's experience"), E ("Encourage treatment and Expedite getting help").[34] This can be a useful tool for health care professionals in assessing and responding to LGBTQ veterans in crisis. Additional VA resources are provided as part of the S.A.V.E. training program.

Safety Planning

Safety plans are developed collaboratively with the LGBTQ veterans to support them through periods of crisis and reduce future risk for suicide.[32,35–37] Safety plans should include 6 components: identification of warning signs, internal coping mechanisms, social supports to engage with to distract from the crisis, social supports to seek out for help, mental health professionals to contact for support, and reduced access to lethal means.[35–37] Health care professionals at the VA have access to a standardized safety planning tool incorporating these 6 components. Veterans are given a copy of the safety plan to use when experiencing worsening psychiatric symptoms or times of crisis.[35] Individuals who are in distress can often be impulsive, and safety plans and restricted access to lethal means have shown to reduce the likelihood of engaging in behaviors that would potentially lead to suicide death.[38] Stanley and colleagues[35] conducted a study and found that 61% of the veterans who endorsed the utilization of the safety plan decrease their risk of suicide. An important part of maintaining the safety of the LBGTQ veterans is to support and provide them with additional resources that can be incorporated into their safety plans. Suggested resources include but are not limited to:

National Suicide Prevention Hotline: 1 to 800 to 273 to 8225
Veteran crisis line: 1 to 800 to 273 to 8255, press 1 or text 838,255
Crisis Text Line: 741,741
LGBTQ hotline: 1 to 888 to 843 to 4564

A free mobile app, the Stanley-Brown Safety Plan,[39] is available to veterans and the general population. It allows for immediate access and frequent updates of their safety plan with internal links to crisis phone numbers.

Restrict Access to Lethal Means

Suicide attempts are often impulsive; therefore, restricted access to lethal means is an important suicide prevention intervention.[38,40] Health care providers should talk to

LGBTQ veterans about the increased risk associated with access to firearms, illicit substances, and alcohol, as well as ways to mitigate risk.[40] Interventions to mitigate firearm risk include installing trigger locks, using a gun safe, storing ammunition separately from the firearm, and giving firearm to a friend, family member, local police, or licensed firearms dealer to store while an individual is at increased risk for suicide.[40,41] Interventions to mitigate risk associated with alcohol and illicit substances include discussing the impact of these substances on judgment, involving the family in safety planning, and connecting the veteran to substance use treatment.[32,40]

Psychological

While there is a need for future research regarding evidence-based treatment of suicidality specifically within the LGBTQ population, there are several psychological treatment modalities for suicidality in the general population supported by randomized controlled trials. Cognitive Behavioral Therapy for Suicide Prevention (CBT-SP) has been found to reduce suicidal behavior in adults when CBT-SP sessions are specifically focused on these behaviors.[5,32,38] CBT-SP is a short-term therapy consisting of an average of 10 to 12 sessions. The sessions are grouped into three phases (**Table 2**).[42]

Dialectical Behavioral Therapy (DBT) was originally developed to decrease self-injurious and suicidal behaviors in patients with borderline personality disorder and is the most studied psychological intervention for suicidal behavior.[43] DBT typically consists of individual psychotherapy, group skills sessions, phone consultation, and a therapist consultation team.[43] During DBT treatment, patients learn about mindfulness, interpersonal effectiveness, emotional regulation, and distress tolerance.[43] Although primarily studied for the treatment of borderline personality disorder, more recent studies have found DBT to significantly reduce suicidal behaviors when compared with usual treatment when applied to other populations.[5,32,38,44,45]

Problem-solving therapy (PST) is a type of CBT developed to enhance patients' coping mechanisms for stressful situations.[32] PST teaches individuals to use problem-solving techniques to avoid self-harm behaviors. It has been found to be beneficial for veterans experiencing suicidal ideation.[32] PST helps veterans to develop coping mechanisms and use the skills learned to improve their quality of life.[32,46]

Pharmacologic

For patients experiencing symptoms of depression, antidepressants have been found to decrease suicidality in adults over the age of 25.[38] Selective serotonin reuptake inhibitors (SSRIs) are typically the first-line antidepressants prescribed due to their effectiveness, side effect profile, and low risk for fatality when taken in overdose.[47] One study analyzed data from 26 countries and found that the number of prescriptions for SSRIs was inversely correlated with the countries' suicide rates.[38] When prescribing antidepressants to suicidal patients, it is critical to know which medications can be lethal if taken in overdose, for example, tricyclic antidepressants are more lethal in overdose than SSRIs.[47]

For patients diagnosed with bipolar disorder, lithium has been found to be an effective monotherapy for mood stabilization. It is the only mood stabilizer that has been found to be protective against suicide in bipolar and unipolar depression.[32,38] In patients diagnosed with schizophrenia and schizoaffective disorder, clozapine is not only an effective medication for psychotic symptoms but has also been found to decrease suicidal ideation and attempts when compared with other antipsychotics.[24,38] Of note, clozapine carries risk for several adverse effects including

Table 2
Cognitive-behavioral therapy for suicide prevention

Phase 1	Phase 2	Phase 3
• Assess safety risk • Establish a treatment plan • Develop a collaborative crisis response plan • Begin developing skills in emotion regulation and crisis management	• Identify thought patterns that contribute to suicidal ideation and behavior • Challenge maladaptive beliefs	• Relapse prevention exercises • Reinforce learned skills

Data from Bryan CJ. Cognitive behavioral therapy for suicide prevention (CBT-SP): Implications for meeting standard of care expectations with suicidal patients. Behav Sci Law. May 2019;37(3):247-258.

neutropenia and myocarditis.[48] It is, therefore, essential to weigh the risks and benefits when prescribing this medication.

Other options for acute suicidality include electroconvulsive therapy (ECT) and ketamine treatment. ECT is a treatment that produces generalized seizures while patients are under general anesthesia.[49] While ECT is highly stigmatized, it has been found to be safe and effective for the treatment of suicidality, severe depression, and bipolar disorder.[49] Ketamine is an anesthetic and has been found to have immediate effects on depressive symptoms and suicidal ideation in unipolar and bipolar depression. It is important to consider that ketamine is a shorter acting medication that also poses abuse potential.[32,38]

VETERANS AFFAIRS-SPECIFIC LESBIAN, GAY, BISEXUAL, TRANSGENDER, AND QUEER RESOURCES

Health care professionals within the VA have more training and experience providing culturally sensitive care to the veteran population.[50] LGBTQ veterans who are actively connected to the larger veteran community have been found to have lower prevalence of suicidal ideation.[5]

The VA Office of Mental Health and Suicide Prevention collaborated with the LGBTQ Health Program to highlight the importance of asking about sexual orientation, gender identity, and preferred pronouns during health care visits to normalize and empower veterans to feel comfortable discussing these topics with their provider.[51] Asking about LGBTQ identities also conveys dignity and respect, and helps the provider to understand the veteran's life and connect them to the most relevant services.

VA facilities have LGBTQ Veteran Care Coordinators who help veterans access the care they need.[52] Care coordinators answer veteran questions, provide information about veteran rights and policies for health care access, advocate for culturally sensitive care, direct veterans to specific services, and help veterans navigate reporting complaints or concerns related to their health care.[52] Services and information available for LGBTQ veterans include gender-affirming hormone and speech therapy, trans-health e-consults, research specific to the LGBTQ population, substance use treatment, treatment and prevention of sexually transmitted infections, support for individuals who have experienced intimate partner violence and military sexual trauma, and mental health care.[52] Furthermore, there are resources available for veterans who have questions about coming out to their provider and finding providers who specialize in LGBTQ health.[52]

SUMMARY

An adequate and comprehensive assessment of suicide risk in LGBTQ veterans requires careful examination of the numerous protective and risk factors that contribute to suicidal ideation, intent, and behavior. It is essential that health care professionals conduct an effective risk analysis using an intersectional lens, a thorough understanding of epidemiology, and the use of evidence-based assessment tools. Suicide risk is an important clinical challenge in the LGBTQ veteran population; a population that is often inequitably served.[53] Resources and expertise are available within the VA health care system; a system that has prioritized providing culturally sensitive, veteran-centric care that addresses the unique needs of the LGBTQ veteran population. For LGBTQ veterans who choose to pursue care outside of the VA health care system, coordination of care between their primary care, mental health care, and VA provider, if there is one, is essential to the achievement of optimal clinical outcomes. Accurately identifying suicide risk factors is the first step in developing a recommended course of treatment that promotes healing and prevents further psychological and physiologic injury.

CLINICS CARE POINTS

- Suicide risk assessment should be completed at every visit.
- Individuals who complete and use their safety plans have a decrease risk of suicide.
- Provide suicide prevention resources to everyone at every visit.

DISCLOSURE

All authors have no commercial or financial conflicts to disclose.

The contents of this article do not represent the views of the Department of Veterans Affairs or the US government. The views expressed here are those of the authors and do not necessarily reflect the position or policy of the United States (US) Department of Veterans Affairs or the US government.

REFERENCES

1. Center for Disease Control and Prevention. Suicide prevention: facts about suicide. Available at: https://www.cdc.gov/suicide/facts/index.html. Accessed on October 22, 2021.
2. Suicide worldwide in 2019: global health estimates. Geneva: World Health Organization; 2021. Available at: https://www.who.int/publications/i/item/9789240026643. Accessed on October 20, 2021.
3. Center for Disease Control and Prevention. Disparities in suicide. Available at: https://www.cdc.gov/suicide/facts/disparities-in-suicide.html. Accessed on December 25, 2021.
4. Suicide awareness voices of education. LGBTQ adults. Available at: https://save.org/lgbtq-resources/lgbtq-adults/. Accessed on December 21, 2021.
5. Tucker RP. Suicide in Transgender veterans: prevalence, prevention, and implications of current policy. Perspect Psychol Sci 2019;14(3):452–68.
6. Department of Veteran's Affairs. National veteran suicide prevention annual report.2021. 2021. Available at: https://www.mentalhealth.va.gov/docs/data-

sheets/2021/2021-National-Veteran-Suicide-Prevention-Annual-Report-FINAL-9-8-21.pdf. Accessed on December 25, 2021.

7. Centers for Disease Control and Prevention, National Center for Injury Prevention and Control. CDC. Web-based injury statistics query and reporting system (WISQARS). 2020. Available at: https://www.cdc.gov/injury/wisqars/. Accessed on October 22, 2021.
8. American Foundation for Suicide Prevention. Suicide data: United States. 2021. Available at: https://www.datocms-assets.com/12810/1616589783-14155afspnationalfactsheet2021m1v2.pdf. Accessed on December 24, 2021.
9. United Health Foundation. America's health rankings. public health impact: suicide. Available at: https://www.americashealthrankings.org/explore/annual/measure/Suicide/state/ALL. Accessed on December 28, 2021.
10. Substance Abuse and Mental Health Services Administration, U.S. Department of Health and Human Services. 2019 National survey on drug use and health: lesbian, gay, & bisexual (LGB) adults. Available at: https://www.samhsa.gov/data/sites/default/files/reports/rpt31104/2019NSDUH-LGB/LGB%202019%20NSDUH.pdf. Accessed on December 29, 2021.
11. American Foundation for Suicide Prevention. Suicide statistics. Available at: https://afsp.org/suicide-statistics/. Accessed on December 24, 2021.
12. Crenshaw K. Demarginalizing the intersection of race and sex: a black feminist critique of antidiscrimination doctrine, feminist theory and antiracist politics. Univ Chicago Leg Forum 1989;1(8):139–67.
13. Crenshaw K. Mapping the margins: intersectionality, identity politics, and violence against women of color. Stanford Law Rev 1990;43:1241.
14. Dallocchio M. Women veterans: examining identity through an intersectional lens. J Mil Veteran Fam Health 2021;7(s1):111–21.
15. Brownstone LM, Holliman BD, Gerber HR, et al. The phenomenology of military sexual trauma among women veterans. Psychol Women Q 2018;42(4):399–413.
16. Department of Veterans Affairs. Military sexual trauma (MST) screening report, fiscal year 2020. 2021. Available at: https://sapr.mil/reports. Accessed January 3, 2022.
17. Lehavot K, Goldberg SB, Chen JA, et al. Do trauma type, stressful life events, and social support explain women veterans' high prevalence of PTSD? Soc Psychiatry Psychiatr Epidemiol 2018;53(9):943–53.
18. Compton MT, Shim RS. The social determinants of mental health. FOC 2015; 13(4):419–25.
19. Sederer LI. The social determinants of mental health. Psychiatr Serv 2016;67(2): 234–5.
20. Tillman S. Protecting our Patients from sexual assault. J Psychosoc Nurs Ment Health Serv 2018;56(3):2–4.
21. Cannon C, Buttell F. Research-supported recommendations for treating LGBTQ perpetrators of IPV: implications for policy and practice. Partner Abuse 2020; 11(4):485–504.
22. National Academies of Sciences, Engineering, and Medicine. Communities in action: pathways to health equity. Washington, DC: The National Academies Press; 2017. Available at: https://www.nap.edu/catalog/24624/communities-in-action-pathways-to-health-equity. Accessed December 27, 2021.
23. Suicide Awareness Voices of Education. Warning signs of suicide. 2021. Available at: https://save.org/about-suicide/warning-signs-risk-factors-protective-factors/. Accessed November 16, 2021.

24. Matsuno E, Israel T. Psychological interventions promoting resilience among transgender individuals: transgender resilience intervention model (TRIM). Couns Psychol 2018;46(5):632–55.
25. Livingston NA, Berke DS, Ruben MA, et al. Experiences of trauma, discrimination, microaggressions, and minority stress among trauma-exposed LGBT veterans: Unexpected findings and unresolved service gaps. Psychol Trauma 2019; 11(7):695–703.
26. Meyer IH. Prejudice, social stress, and mental health in lesbian, gay, and bisexual populations: conceptual issues and research evidence. Psychol Bull 2003; 129(5):674–97.
27. Levenson JS, Craig SL, Austin A. Trauma-informed and affirmative mental health practices with LGBTQ+ clients. [published online ahead of print] 2021 Apr 15]. Psychol Serv 2021;1–11.
28. Goldbach JT, Rhoades H, Green D, et al. Is there a need for LGBT-specific suicide crisis services? Crisis 2019;40(3):203–8.
29. Shipherd JC, Ruben MA, Livingston NA, et al. Treatment experiences among LGBT veterans with discrimination-based trauma exposure: a pilot study. J Trauma Dissociation 2018;19(4):461–75.
30. King CA, Horwitz A, Czyz E, et al. Suicide risk screening in healthcare settings: identifying males and females at risk. J Clin Psychol Med Settings 2017; 24(1):8–20.
31. Bahraini N, Brenner LA, Barry C, et al. Assessment of rates of suicide risk screening and prevalence of positive screening results among us veterans after implementation of the veterans affairs suicide risk identification Strategy. JAMA Netw Open 2020;3(10):e2022531.
32. Department of Veterans Affairs, Department of Defense. VA/DoD clinical practice guideline for the assessment and management of patients at risk for suicide. Available at: https://www.healthquality.va.gov/guidelines/MH/srb/VADoDSuicideRiskFullCPGFinal5088212019.pdf. Accessed January 5, 2022.
33. Suicide Prevention Resource Center; U.S. Department of Health and Human Services, Substance Abuse and Mental Health Services Administration, Center for Mental Health Services. Available at: https://www.sprc.org/resources-programs/operation-save-va-suicide-prevention-gatekeeper-training. Accessed December 28, 2021.
34. U.S. Department of Veteran Affairs. VA S.A.V.E. Training. Supporting our veterans. Available at: https://www.mentalhealth.va.gov/mentalhealth/suicide_prevention/docs/VA_SAVE_Training.pdf. Accessed on December 28, 2021.
35. Stanley B, Chaudhury SR, Chesin M, et al. An emergency department intervention and follow-up to reduce suicide risk in the va: acceptability and effectiveness. Psychiatr Serv 2016;67(6):680–3.
36. Suicide and serious mental illness: an overview of considerations, assessment, and safety planning | suicide prevention resource center. Available at: https://sprc.org/resources-programs/suicide-serious-mental-illness-overview-considerations-assessment-safety-planning. Accessed January 6, 2022.
37. U.S Department of Veteran Affairs. Veteran Health Administration. Office for suicide prevention. veteran outreach toolkit preventing veteran suicide is everyone's business a community call to action. Available at: https://www.va.gov/ve/docs/outreachToolkitPreventingVeteranSuicideIsEveryonesBusiness.pdf. Accessed on January 6, 2022.
38. Turecki G, Brent DA. Suicide and suicidal behaviour. Lancet 2016;387(10024): 1227–39.

39. Stanley-Brown safety plan. Version 2.7. Troy, NY. Two Penguins Studios LLC.
40. Harvard School of Public Health. Means matter. Available at: https://www.hsph.harvard.edu/means-matter/recommendations/clinicians/. Accessed January 5, 2022.
41. Allchin A, Chaplin V, Horwitz J. Limiting access to lethal means: applying the social ecological model for firearm suicide prevention. Inj Prev 2019;25(Suppl 1):i44–8.
42. Bryan CJ. Cognitive behavioral therapy for suicide prevention (CBT-SP): Implications for meeting standard of care expectations with suicidal patients. Behav Sci Law 2019;37(3):247–58.
43. May JM, Richardi TM, Barth KS. Dialectical behavior therapy as treatment for borderline personality disorder. Ment Health Clin 2016;6(2):62–7.
44. Goodman M, Banthin D, Blair NJ, et al. A randomized trial of dialectical behavior therapy in high-risk suicidal veterans. J Clin Psychiatry 2016;77(12):e1591–600.
45. DeCou CR, Comtois KA, Landes SJ. Dialectical behavior therapy is effective for the treatment of suicidal behavior: a meta-analysis. Behav Ther 2019;50(1):60–72.
46. Cuijpers P, de Wit L, Kleiboer A, et al. Problem-solving therapy for adult depression: an updated meta-analysis. Eur Psychiatry 2018;48:27–37.
47. Rush J. Unipolar major depression in adults: choosing initial treatment. Available at: https://www.uptodate.com/contents/unipolar-major-depression-in-adults-choosing-initial-treatment?search=depression%20treatment&source=search_result&selectedTitle=1~150&usage_type=default&display_rank=1. Accessed December 21, 2021.
48. Scott Stroup SM. Schizophrenia in adults: Maintenance therapy and side effect management. Available at: https://www.uptodate.com/contents/schizophrenia-in-adults-maintenance-therapy-and-side-effect-management?search=schizophrenia%20treatment&source=search_result&selectedTitle=1~150&usage_type=default&display_rank=1. Accessed December 21, 2021.
49. Kellner C. Overview of electroconvulsive therapy (ECT) for adults. Available at: https://www.uptodate.com/contents/overview-of-electroconvulsive-therapy-ect-for-adults?search=electroconvulsive%20therapy&source=search_result&selectedTitle=1~120&usage_type=default&display_rank=1lskdflkdjs. Accessed December 21, 2021.
50. Tanielian T, Farris C, Batka C, et al. Ready to serve: community-based provider capacity to deliver culturally competent, quality mental health care to veterans and their families. RAND Corporation; 2014. Available at: https://www.rand.org/content/dam/rand/pubs/research_reports/RR800/RR806/RAND_RR806.pdf. Accessed December 20, 2021.
51. U.S. Department of Veteran Affairs. Sharing LGBTQ+ identity with providers. make the connection. Available at: https://www.maketheconnection.net/events/sharing-LGBTQ-identity-with-providers/. Accessed January 5, 2022.
52. U.S. Department of Veterans Affairs. LGBTQ+ health program. Available at: https://www.patientcare.va.gov/LGBT/index.asp. Accessed December 21, 2021.
53. Kondo K, Low A, Everson T, et al. Health disparities in veterans: a map of the evidence. Med Care 2017;55(Suppl 9 Suppl 2):S9–15.

Caring for Veteran Women

Collaborative Nursing Approaches to Improve Care

Anna Strewler, MS, AGPCNP-BC[a,*], Keisha Bellamy, MSN, MBA, NE-BC[b]

KEYWORDS

- Veteran women • Strength-based nursing • Communication skills

KEY POINTS

- Use a strength-based approach when caring for Veteran women in health care settings.
- Use trauma-informed health care practices during interpersonal collaboration and system-level improvements.
- Recognize, honor, and individualize care to the intersecting identities of Veteran women.
- Adopt holistic models of care to enhance a sense of community belonging for Veteran women.
- Embrace opportunities, when possible, to offer participation in research to Veteran women to ultimately improve the care provided to this population.

Women represent the fastest-growing group among Veterans in the United States and are projected to comprise 18% of the Veteran population by 2040.[1] Although women have been serving informally in the military since 1775, they officially could enter the Army Nurse Corps in 1901, and since 2016, all military positions have been open to women. They represent a highly successful group, having obtained, for example, higher numbers of bachelors and advanced degrees than their non-Veteran counterparts.[1] However, despite these military and postmilitary achievements, many clinical resources for nurses and clinicians caring for Veteran women focus on screening for and treating the disabling medical and psychosocial conditions facing this population, such as military sexual trauma (MST), post-traumatic stress disorder (PTSD), musculoskeletal conditions, and migraines. Although these resources provide critical guidance for clinicians in both Veterans Health Administration (VHA) and non-VHA settings,[2,3] the goal of this article is to complement them with a strength-based approach to improve the overall experience of health care for Veteran women.

[a] San Francisco VA Health Care System, University of California, San Francisco, 4150 Clement Street, San Francisco, CA 94121, USA; [b] San Francisco VA Health Care System, 4150 Clement Street, San Francisco, CA 94121, USA

* Corresponding author.

E-mail address: anna.strewler@va.gov

Nurs Clin N Am 57 (2022) 359–373
https://doi.org/10.1016/j.cnur.2022.04.004
0029-6465/22/Published by Elsevier Inc.

Our theoretic framework is Laurie N. Gottlieb's strength-based nursing (SBN), which emphasizes the unique role of the nurse to promote "empowerment, self-efficacy, and hope" when caring for patients and families.[4] Composed of eight core values (**Box 1**), Gottlieb's framework charges nurses with recognizing, eliciting, and drawing on the "inner and outer" strengths of a person, their family, and community to foster health and healing as a complement to biomedical, disease-focused approaches to health care.[4] Veteran women, with their vast degree of diversity, experience, resilience, and professional and life skills and training, deserve an approach to their care that recognizes and honors these strengths while assisting with healing from their unique health challenges. Using an SBN approach leads to care that is individualized and focuses on the interpersonal aspects of partnering with and providing care for Veteran women, improving not only health outcomes but also health care experience.

Using this lens, we aim to focus on four key areas unique to Veteran women that provide opportunities for nurses and clinicians to improve this population's health care experience by highlighting both their strengths and challenges and using specific interpersonal skills. Given the high rate of premilitary, military, and postmilitary trauma exposure among Veteran women, we will first describe trauma-informed health care practices to complement medical assessments and treatments for histories of trauma and sequela, such as PTSD. Next, we describe the strengths and challenges of Veteran women according to some of the intersectional identities they hold and offer practice recommendations for identity-affirming and more equitable health care. Then, we highlight evidence-based resources and health care approaches that are person-affirming and promote a sense of belonging for Veteran women in health care. Finally, we suggest approaches for nurses and clinicians to ethically increase the participation of Veteran women in research to further improve care for this population.

A final note on our definition of this population for the purpose of this article should make explicit to readers that we define Veteran women to comprise any Veteran who self-identifies with the term "woman," regardless of sex assigned at birth. This includes transgender women in addition to intersex and gender nonconforming and nonbinary Veterans (we use the terms transgender and gender diverse [TGD]) who identify fully or partially, now or in the past or future, as women. The National Transgender Discrimination Survey estimates that approximately 134,300 (19%) of the transgender population in the United States are actively serving or historically served in the military.[5] In fact, transgender individuals are more likely to serve in the military than cisgender individuals, which results in their overrepresentation in the Veteran

Box 1
Strength-based nursing: eight-core values[4]

1. Health and healing
2. Uniqueness
3. Holism and embodiment
4. Subjective reality and created meaning
5. Person and environment are integral
6. Self-determination
7. Learning, timing, and readiness
8. Collaborative partnership

population.[6] In each of the four aforementioned discussion sections, we make efforts to include literature (when available) and clinical recommendations that are gender-inclusive.

DISCUSSION

Experiences of Trauma

In this section, we aim to emphasize a lifespan approach to understanding the impact of trauma on Veteran women and recommend specific nursing practices to support the care of Veteran women with trauma experiences.

Strengths

In terms of strengths to recognize, social support and "hardiness" were found to be predictors of improved mental health, lessened severity of PTSD, and alcohol and drug use among a large female and diverse sample of recently returned Veterans, highlighting the importance of both innate characteristics and social networks in promoting resilience and health.[7] Identifying, naming, and incorporating individual Veteran's strengths in these areas are critical to ensuring quality care and are incorporated into our practice recommendations as follows.

Challenges

The prevalence of trauma in the premilitary, during service, and postmilitary periods is noticeable. Researchers have recently called for better screening and treatment of *pre*-military trauma and abuse in active-duty servicewomen because of their high rates and correlation with the eventual development of PTSD and disability.[8,9] Trauma exposures during the military may include combat-related trauma, MST, intimate partner violence, and others. MST is experienced by around 38.4% of Veteran women[10] and is strongly associated with the development of PTSD, chronic physical symptoms, cardiovascular risk factors, weight loss, and hypothyroidism.[11] PTSD accounts for the highest percentage of service-connected disabilities for women Veterans at 11.8%.[1] As an especially vulnerable population, 75% of unhoused Veteran women report combat-related trauma and are three times more likely to have experienced MST than housed Veteran women.[12] The prevalence of traumatic experiences *after* military service is also higher for Veteran women than men.[13] Astonishingly, the adjusted odds ratio of MST was 2.73, and the diagnosis of PTSD was 2.82 for transgender Veterans (not further broken down by specific gender identity) compared with non-transgender Veterans.[14]

Practice recommendations

To complement the trauma-related screening and treatment recommendations that are well described in the literature[2] and in VHA treatment guides (otherwise known as trauma-specific services that are critical for nurses as well as medical colleagues to use), we aim to provide a framework for improved everyday communication and interpersonal practices and institutional processes to improve the overall health care experience for Veteran women: trauma-informed care. The Substance Abuse and Mental Health Services Administration's (SAMHSA, 2014) definition of a trauma-informed approach is:

> A program, organization, or system that is trauma-informed realizes the widespread impact of trauma and understands potential paths for recovery; recognizes the signs and symptoms of trauma in clients, families, staff, and others involved in the system; and responds by fully integrating knowledge about trauma into policies, procedures, and practices, and seeks to actively resist re-traumatization.[15]

Its core principles include physical and psychological safety, trustworthiness, collaboration, empowerment, and appreciation of the patient's intersecting personal identities and historical contexts[15] and are well aligned with nursing practice. Although a key tenet of trauma-informed care is to assume a history of trauma and consider these practices as "universal precautions," given the high rates and health consequences of trauma in the Veteran women population, using this approach is especially critical. **Box 2** outlines the specific trauma-informed clinical practices for Veteran women.

Intersectionality

We know that Veteran status alone may confer stressors and mental and physical health conditions and, according to Veteran critical theory, unique disadvantages, oppression, marginalization, and negative stereotypes.[18] Here, we aim to additionally highlight other non-Veteran identities held by Veteran women (such as race, ethnicity, gender, sexuality, and so forth) and the ways these uniquely combine on an individual level to influence both negative and positive experiences, health outcomes, and practice considerations. We base this section on the intersectionality theory, first described by Kimberlé Crenshaw,[19] which recognizes the interdependence of

Box 2
Trauma-informed health care practices for Veteran women

Offer and actively improve health care system intake processes to be more simple, clear, gender identity-affirming, and welcoming.

Use a trauma-informed approach as a universal standard of care for all patients. Assume, before even asking, about experiences of trauma.[12]

Before beginning, ask whether the patient has preferences around the health care encounter: "Is there anything I/we can do to make this visit feel safe and comfortable for you? What has worked well in the past?"

Continually explain and ask permission before and throughout every step of a clinical encounter: check-in, rooming, vitalization, history-taking, physical examination, procedures, and providing education and recommendations.

Accept declination throughout the encounter.

Use nonjudgmental, positive, identity-affirming, and professional language.[16]

Ensure privacy and offer chaperone/companion support (offer this privately).[16]

Ask broadly, in a non-triggering way, how stressful life events may be playing a role in a patient's health or experience of health care: "We know that stressful life events can affect people's health and well-being. Is there anything you think I should know about your personal history that might be affecting your health today?"

Offer to connect patients to trauma-specific treatment services. Help facilitate timely access to this care and all other referrals through team-based care coordination.[16]

Collaborate with and empower patients to guide plans of care.[12]

Identify, verbalize, and capitalize on patient strengths. Encourage self-care strategies. Set health goals that are specific, measurable, achievable, realistic, and time-bound.[16]

Identify and connect patient with additional support systems (health care-based interdisciplinary, holistic care [ie, Whole Health],[16] and community-based resources).[17]

Ask for feedback on health care services provided to do your practice and setting more collaborative and safer.[16]

identities to inform differential experiences and power, privilege, systemic and interpersonal oppression, and access to resources. Also, helpfully, the minority stress model, developed to describe the experience of lesbian, gay, and bisexual people (and more recently applied to TGD individuals), similarly recognizes stress factors in this population but importantly also resilience factors, which we hope to highlight as well.[20] Most studies on Veteran women examine intersectionality between gender, race/ethnicity, and sexuality.

Strengths

Veterans represent a racially diverse population, with a quarter currently holding ethnic/racial minority identities, and are anticipated to reach a third over the next 2 decades.[21] Actually, *more* women Veterans in the United States hold ethnic/racial and/or sexual minority identities than their non-Veteran counterparts.[22] By the same token that intersectionality posits compounding structural disadvantages with multiple marginalized identities, an argument can be made for compounding resiliency and protective factors.[23] In a 2019 study, for example, women Veterans who identified as both racial/ethnic and sexual minorities had lower rates of depression, anxiety, and sexist events than their heterosexual counterparts. Hypotheses to explain these results include the development of protective and affirming communities, effective coping behaviors, and a sense of unity and purpose in the face of disadvantage and discrimination.[22] These findings caution us from assuming a solely challenge-based narrative and remind us to elicit and support areas of strength in Veteran women.

Challenges

To equitize health and well-being among Veteran women, we must also recognize the ways in which multiple marginalized identities confer risk of poor health outcomes because of structural oppression. Examples include higher PTSD symptoms among racial/ethnic minority Veteran women and increased depression, anxiety, sexist events, and less social support reported by racial/ethnic minority heterosexual women compared with White Veteran women.[22] We also see Black and Hispanic-identified Veteran women more likely to report diabetes than White Veteran women, American Indian and Hispanic women less likely to use mental health resources, Asian Pacific Islander (API) Veteran women more likely to screen positive for PTSD, and LGBT (Lesbian, Gay, Bisexual, and Transgender) Veteran women more likely to report alcohol overuse and smoking than heterosexual Veteran women.[22,24] Of note, one recent study found less receipt of brief intervention among Black and API Veterans with women unhealthy alcohol use compared with White women despite universal screening and treatment resources in the VHA system.[25] This disparity, in particular, leads us to recognize the effect not only of compounding structural oppression in these populations but also the effect of (often unconscious) bias and inequitable treatment by health care systems and providers.

Practice recommendations

Although no one-size-fits-all approach exists, **Box 3** presents the best practices to consider when serving Veteran women in a way that honors their multiple identities while seeking to recognize strengths and remit health disparities.

Sense of Belonging in Veteran Community

In this section, we discuss caring for women Veterans in the context of their connection to the health care system and the larger Veteran community. As policy changes continue to evolve, the presence of women Veterans continues to expand. As mentioned in our introduction, although women have been informally serving in the

Box 3
Health care practices in recognition of Veteran women's intersectional identities

Introduce yourself with name, role, and gender pronouns.

Use gender-neutral terms to address a patient until their self-stated gender identity is shared. Ask what name and pronouns a patient uses in a private setting. Use it consistently.

Use a strength-based, open-ended approach to ask about, rather than assuming identities (i.e. as recommended to undergraduate medical students by Davis and colleagues [2021, p. 3]):

- *"I've learned that people's backgrounds have a great deal to do with health ... I'd like to hear whatever you feel comfortable telling me about what you feel proud of related to* [one or more of your identities]*."*
- *"What might you feel comfortable sharing with me about a challenge you've had related to your* [identities]*."*[26]

Acknowledge your own identities and areas of power/privileges/oppression, especially when a patient's identities differ from one or more of your own.

Consistently elicit patients' areas of pride and success.[27]

Elicit and mobilize health care and community resources to address psychosocial barriers.

Offer interpreter services when needed.

Offer the option of identity-concordant providers, team members, and peer support when available.

Engage in shared decision-making throughout the treatment planning to inform individualized, aligned, and identity-affirming care.

Engage in population health and systems improvement to identify populations who may benefit from enhanced services, preventative efforts, and resource allocation to improve health outcomes and reduce disparities.

Engage in training and continuous, dedicated practice in cultural humility, remedying social/structural inequities,[22] relationship-centered communication,[26] and upstander skills and behaviors.

military much longer, it was not until 1901 that their presence was formally acknowledged. Moreover, it was only in 1948 that servicewomen were granted full Veteran status.[28] In 1975, women were allowed to serve in combat positions, which resulted in an increased number of women who serve in the military[29] and subsequently those who are eligible to receive care in the VHA. Although not all may be eligible for VHA services, there are approximately 2 million women Veterans, with only an estimated 740,000 receiving care in the VHA.[30] It is important for nurses and clinicians to recognize that not all Veterans will receive care through the VHA and may not be aware of benefits for which they are eligible.

Strengths

It is critical to emphasize that despite less than half of eligible Veteran women seeking health care and perhaps other benefits from the Department of Veterans Affairs, this population, compared with their civilian counterparts, is thriving. Moreover, the lack of specific communities/organizations (such as Veteran Service Organizations) that are devoted exclusively to women Veterans in comparison to their overall achievements is astounding. Specifically, their collective achievements include higher levels of education, lower rates of poverty, and higher median household incomes than their non-Veteran counterparts.[1] One could posit that given their socioeconomic and educational success, there may be less need for Veteran women to seek engagement with VHA services compared with their male Veteran counterparts.

Challenges

Historically, the general population is less likely to think of women as Veterans,[28] which may discourage them from seeking care in the VHA. We know that women who *do* identify strongly with their Veteran identity and hold positive regard for it are more likely to feel as though they "fit" in the VHA system and to access services to which they are entitled.[28] However, anecdotally, it is possible that women's Veteran identity is not as tied to their sense of self as it is for Veteran men. At VHA facilities, it is common to see Veteran men wearing a t-shirt, jacket, and/or hat that identifies their military branch (eg, Army, Navy, Air Force, Marine Corps, Coast Guard) and era of service (eg, WWII, Korea, Vietnam, Cold War/Peace Time, Gulf War, Post-9/11) as well as any accomplishments earned during their time in the military. In contrast, it is rare for Veteran women to display similar identifying attire that connects them to the Veteran community—they seem to hide in plain sight. It is the responsibility of each VHA and non-VHA health care organization to create an environment of inclusion and safety for Veteran women.

Overall, women Veterans' least positive perceptions of VHA care were the availability and logistics of needed services for gynecologic and other female sex-specific procedures (ie, mammography and pregnancy-related care).[31] In 2014, VHA introduced the Veterans Choice Program (VCP) to expand timely access to medical care for Veterans by the way of contracting care to non-VHA organizations.[32] Regarding female sex-specific and gynecologic care, Veterans reported experiencing challenges (eg, scheduling VCP appointments, timely sharing of VCP care results, and unpaid VCP bills) related to VCP that were equally problematic as accessing and receiving timely care in VHA.[32] Contracting gynecologic and other female sex-specific care to the community may alienate women Veterans from seeking VHA care.

It is important to communicate the scope of the barriers experienced by all women Veterans, including LGBT and gender diverse Veterans. Nonheterosexual women are more likely to report feeling unwelcome and unsafe due to harassment by male veterans at VHA as being of greatest concern.[33] The barriers to accessing VHA care expressed by these women were thought to be mitigated by the VHAs "zero-tolerance standard for harassment of any kind." However, there are instances when the intent of the policy fails to be upheld, and more education (to providers and Veterans) is needed to facilitate timely reporting.[5] Although the legislation impacting transgender service members has vacillated between acceptance and support to direct rejection and opposition, the Department of Defense (DoD) has most recently settled on support for gender transition of transgender service members during military service,[34] reflecting a more open policy. Our hope is that a more accepting DoD will eventually extend to a better health care experience for TGD Veterans. In fact, VHA has increased its ability to provide timely care to transgender veterans through its own services and VCP after transgender Veterans reported the following barriers to VHA care: long delays in receiving care, extensive travel to receive care, lack of knowledge about transgender health among providers, and concerns about personal safety/harassment. However, just as cisgender women Veterans' care is often contracted to non-VHA medical organizations, so often is transgender-specific care, such as hormone therapy,[5] resulting in similar potential alienation. Finally, given a higher prevalence of housing instability among transgender Veterans compared with cisgender Veterans,[6] it is especially important for health care systems to offer services to engage this population in care that is inclusive and affirming.

Practice recommendations

VHA adopted the Whole Health (WH) model (**Fig. 1**) with the goal of shifting the dialogue from a medical/disease-orientated system to one of health promotion and

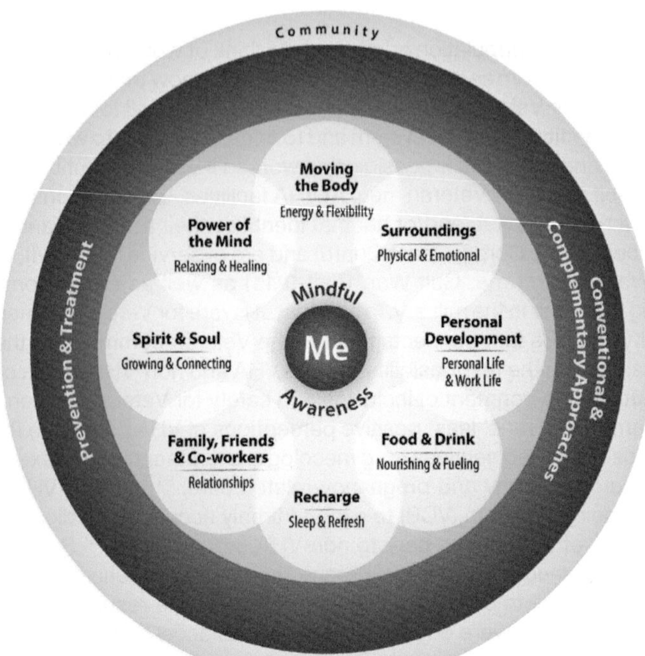

Fig. 1. Whole health wheel. (*From* U. S. Department of Veterans Affairs. Whole Health. The Circle of Health. Available at: https://www.va.gov/WHOLEHEALTH/circle-of-health/index.asp. Accessed December 29, 2021; with permission.)

disease prevention.[35] This is an aspect of VHA care that many community-based providers, as well as some internal VHA health care personnel, may underestimate in its ability to support Veterans in having agency more than their own health and advancing their care based on their personal health care goals. We emphasize this model in this section as a modality for nurses and clinicians to recognize and incorporate all parts of women Veterans' identities and goals into their care to improve their individual sense of belonging in their chosen health care system. The WH model's implementation into care (particularly for those who are currently underserved by health care systems) can result in personalized, empowered, patient-driven discussions about what the individual patient envisions for their health.[35] It is used in the VHA by any trained health care personnel and is also available as formal referrals for more holistically integrated health care services. We also highlight the VHA Women's Health Transition Training (**Box 4**) as a method of self-guided engagement of women Veterans in the larger Veteran community.[36] **Box 5** highlights our recommendations for nurses and clinicians to increase women Veterans' sense of belonging in health care settings, and **Box 6** provides the web-based resources for women seeking to access the Veteran community and VHA care.

Improving Participation in Research

In this section, we address the lack of representation among Veteran women in biomedical research and the adverse impact, and this gap creates in individualized clinical care as well as research. Although there are many clinical trials underway at any given time, women across population groups are less likely to be aware of or

Box 4
VA Women's Health Transition Training—Center for women Veterans[36]

PHASE 1: Shift from Active Duty

PHASE 2: Understanding the VA

PHASE 3: Available Women's Health Services

PHASE 4: Enrolling in VA

PHASE 5: Transition Assistance

participate in clinical research.[41] In addition to discussing the underrepresentation of women Veterans in research, it is important to recognize that the underrepresentation of women service members in research is also of concern.[29] VHA, in conjunction with DoD, has taken up the charge to examine these gaps and increase research to understand and improve health care services for women.[29] Although the barriers to recruiting and retaining military women in research (eg, lengthy deployments, unpredictable military exercises, foreign assignments) differ for Veterans, areas of overlap exist.[29] In 2010, the VHA Women's Health Research Network (WHRN) was created to address knowledge gaps in the evidence related to Veteran women's health and health care.[42] The WHRN prioritized research in the following areas: mental health, primary care and prevention, reproductive health, complex chronic conditions/aging and long-term care, access to care and rural health, and post-deployment health.

Box 5
Increasing Veteran women's sense of belonging in health care settings

Non-VHA health care systems: Offer and actively improve intake systems to identify military service during initial intake.

Ask, before assuming, about current or historical engagement in VHA care.

Before beginning, ask whether the patient has preferences around the health care encounter: "*What matters to you?*"[35] It is also appropriate to inquire before or at the initial intake if Veteran women would like to receive care in women-specific clinic settings.

Continually offer and engage the Whole Health (WH) model, emphasizing personalized, proactive, and patient-driven care.[35] Non-VHA health care systems can share WH informational links: https://www.va.gov/wholehealth/.[37]

Accept declination of services throughout the encounter with the understanding that a formal WH consult can be placed at any time and/or initiation of formal WH care can be a self-referral.

When VCP is used, discuss the logistical process transparently along with timelines for information to be shared between VHA and non-VHA providers.[32]

Thank Veterans for their service.[12]

Identify and connect patients with additional resources/support systems (health care-based interdisciplinary, holistic care [ie, WH],[16] and community-based resources)[17]

Ask for feedback on health care services provided to do your practice and setting more collaborative and safer.[16]

Although the standard of practice at each VHA facility differs when a Veteran does not seem for or consistently cancels appointments, Veteran women and transgender and gender diverse populations may benefit from a nurse or clinician-initiated call to ascertain what, if any, barriers (eg, harassment) to accessing care exist.[33]

Box 6
Web-based resources for women Veterans to connect with others

Create Community. Connect with Other Veterans[38]:
https://www.womenshealth.va.gov/WOMENSHEALTH/connect-with-other-veterans.asp

Directory of State Women Veteran Coordinators[39]:
https://www.naswvc.org/state-coordinators-1/georgia

Women Veterans Network[40]:
https://www.wovenwomenvets.org/

Strengths

Successful examples of inclusion in research are the Million Veteran Program (MVP) and the All of Us (AoU) studies. MVP is a national research program that was launched in 2011 to learn how genes, lifestyle, and military exposures affect health and illness. It is one of the world's largest programs on genetics and health, with more than 850,000 Veterans enrolled and women Veterans represent approximately 75,600 (9%) of enrolled Veterans.[43,44]

Although AoU was not primarily designed for the Veteran population, Veterans are a unique population for whom specialized recruitment efforts have been implemented. The AoU research program is similar to MVP in that it focuses on the intersection of environment, lifestyle, and biology with a goal of recruiting a million research participants from populations that have historically been underrepresented in biomedical research. There is an emphasis placed on the recruitment and retention of diversity in participants, including race, ethnicity, age group, region of the country, gender identity, sexual orientation, socioeconomic status, education, disability, and health status.[45] It is hoped that understanding the health habits of such a large cohort for such an extensive time (10 years) will allow for more patient-centered care tailored to the needs of individuals and subsequently decrease health disparities.

VHA displays strength in mental health research that includes women Veterans. As one might expect, VHA is currently a leader in the field of addressing PTSD.[42] Research and, therefore, literature are available in larger quantities on PTSD and MST than other biomedical challenges facing this population. Another mental health research topic explored in this population is substance abuse. Understanding that women Veterans seek care at the VHA primarily for mental health issues may bias the direction of topics investigated.[46] Sex-specific research topics such as breast cancer and reproductive health have also been researched at a greater frequency than other physical health topics, such as hypertension and diabetes.[42]

There are many successful examples of research, including TGD participants in the context of engagement with HIV programs and funding sources. Less is known about conducting research involving this population regarding other health concerns. Asquith[47] identified the following as motivators to participate in TGD research: facilitating TGD community, research led by TGD researchers, compensating participants, research integrated into routine health care, research with application outside the TGD community, and contributing positively to TGD communities. Although this study did not specifically mention Veterans, its findings may potentially be applied to more inclusive research practices with this Veteran population.

The DoD, VHA, Food and Drug Administration (FDA), and National Institutes of Health (NIH) have all prioritized the advancement of research for women across the lifespan by offering education, successful case studies, strategic plan alignment, and care initiatives that align with opening clinical studies to women to facilitate better understanding and increased health equity.

Challenges

Marginalized groups such as women[29] and TGD Veterans traditionally present with recruitment and retention challenges for biomedical research. Although these groups have significant representation within VHA, conducting interventional research among them has been challenging because of the following: logistics, socioeconomic challenges, small cohorts, lack of diversity among research staff, and inflexible clinic times.[41] VHA systems can cover large geographic areas that often include urban as well as rural locations. The large geographic area can result in logistical and financial burdens for study participants, and assistance with transportation may help mitigate these challenges. Using diverse and identity-concordant research personnel during the recruitment and research processes is critical.[41] Finally, with work and family obligations, it is recommended that clinic hours may be adjusted to allow working, student, and care giving women better support for participation.[41]

It is also of note that although topics such as PTSD and MST have yielded a larger body of scientific work, health concerns such as hypertension, diabetes, depression, and anxiety have not been as thoroughly explored in this population.[42,46] Although their clinical prevalence is high, there is a deficiency in exploring these topics from a primary care and chronic disease perspective. What is consistently lacking in women's Veteran research are randomized-controlled trials (RCTs) and studies on the quality of care.[42,46]

Barriers discussed by TGD study participants in health research by Asquith[47] include the following: distrust/dislike of health care and research settings, non-identification with or narrow definition of gendered labels by researchers, the "cisgender lens" of research, "privacy concerns," inaccessibility and lack of awareness of studies, and "research that is objectifying/exploitive." Although these barriers are representative of one research study, its recommendations for gender identity-affirming research that includes "community engagement and participation, transparency, and trust" (Asquith, 2021) are critical to advancing research and health care for TGD participants—Veteran and non-Veteran alike.[47]

Practice recommendations

As women remain underrepresented in research, one barrier that nurses and clinicians can work to mitigate is the lack of literacy and awareness among Veteran women about clinical trials. The FDA has created a helpful handout to support conversations between health care workers and women patients around participation in health care research.[48] It is also critical that nurses and clinicians increase their knowledge on the importance of recognizing sex and gender differences to improve the provision of health care using available resources[49] and stay abreast of current studies open for their patients' potential enrollment.

SUMMARY

We hope that the discussion sections above build on existing literature to support the health care needs of Veteran women. Certain limitations warrant description. One limitation of this article is that few sources cited provide evidence specifically supporting the use of recommended interpersonal care approaches when caring for Veteran women. Although several recommendations cited are recommended by authors studying best practices in this population, they have not been explicitly compared with other modalities through RCTs to assess their efficacy compared with standard of care. We also acknowledge that these descriptions and recommendations for caring for Veteran women do not represent a comprehensive literature review and as such omit certain health challenges such as homelessness, eating disorders, and gastrointestinal disorders that also profoundly affect this population.

Although it is critical that nurses and clinicians learn assessment and treatment modalities to work with patients experiencing common conditions, such as PTSD, MST, musculoskeletal conditions, and homelessness, it is equally important to emphasize the interpersonal approaches and skills used to do so. This article seeks to describe both strengths and challenges for Veteran women and provides specific recommendations for improving their overall experience of health care. We especially highlight the importance of using a trauma-informed approach, acknowledging and affirming Veteran women's intersectional identities, and assessing and engaging patients holistically to set and work toward self-stated health care goals (ie, the WH model). These approaches hold concepts of autonomy, empowerment, and individualization as paramount and importantly encourage the clinician to partner with patients to elicit and incorporate Veterans' strengths into plans of care. Moreover, these concepts and approaches are especially critical to embody when caring for Veteran women from identity groups that are underserved and/or historically oppressed or inequitably treated in health care (ie, non-White, non-cisgender, and so forth). Finally, we encourage clinicians to engage Veteran women in further research to continuously optimize their care.

CLINICS CARE POINTS

- Use trauma-informed health care practices throughout interpersonal collaboration with Veteran women and make systems-level improvements.
- Recognize, acknowledge, and honor the intersecting identities of Veteran women and offer identity-affirming care to promote patient-aligned wellness and improve health equity.
- Adopt and offer holistic, individualized care plans to enhance acknowledgment and a sense of community belonging for Veteran women in health care settings.
- Offer and facilitate opportunities, when possible, for Veteran women to participate in research to improve overall understanding of and care for this population.

DISCLOSURE

No disclosures.

REFERENCES

1. Department of Veterans Affairs National Center for Veterans Analysis and Statistics. The past, present and future of women veterans. 2017. Available at: https://www.va.gov/vetdata/docs/specialreports/women_veterans_2015_final.pdf. Accessed December 17, 2021.
2. Levander XA, Overland MK. Care of women veterans. Med Clin North America 2015;99(3):651–62.
3. Committee on Health Care for Underserved Women. American College of Obstetricians and Gynecologists. Committee opinion no. 547: Health care for women in the military and women veterans. Obstetrics and gynecology 2012;120(6):1538–42.
4. Gottlieb LN. Strengths-based nursing. Am J Nurs 2014;114(8):24–32.
5. Rosentel K, Hill BJ, Lu C, et al. Transgender veterans and the Veterans Health Administration: exploring the experiences of transgender veterans in the Veterans Affairs healthcare system. Transgender Health 2016;1(1):108–16.

6. Carter SP, Montgomery AE, Henderson ER, et al. Housing instability characteristics among transgender veterans cared for in the Veterans Health Administration: 2013-2016. Am J PublicHealth 2019;109(10):1413–8.
7. Eisen SV, Schultz MR, Glickman ME, et al. Postdeployment resilience as a predictor of mental health in Operation Enduring Fredom/Operation Iraqi Freedom returnees. Am J Preventative Med 2014;47(6):754–61.
8. Zinzow HM, Grubaugh AL, Monnier S, et al. Trauma among female veterans: a critical review. Trauma Violence Abuse 2007;8(4):384–400.
9. Parnell D, Ram V, Cazares P, et al. Sexual assault and disabling PTSD in active duty service women. Mil Med 2018;183(9–10):e481–8.
10. Wilson L. The prevalence of military sexual trauma: a meta-analysis. Trauma, Violence & Abuse 2018;19(5):584–97.
11. Suris A, Lind L. Military sexual trauma: a review of prevalence and associated health consequences in veterans. Trauma, Violence & Abuse 2008;9(4):250–69.
12. Gerber MR. Trauma-informed care of veterans. In: Gerber MR, editor. Trauma-informed healthcare approaches. Cham (Switzerland): Springer; 2019. p. 107–22.
13. Kelley ML, Brancu M, Robbins AT, et al. Drug use and childhood-, military-, and post-military trauma exposure among women and men veterans. Drug and Alcohol Dependence 2015;152:201–8.
14. Brown GR, Jones KT. Mental health and medical health disparities in 5135 transgender veterans receiving healthcare in the Veterans Health Administration: a case-control study. LGBT Health 2016;3(2):122–31.
15. Substance Abuse and Mental Health Services Administration (SAMHSA), SAMHSA's working definition of trauma and principles and guidance for a trauma-informed approach. 2014. SMA 14-4884. Accessed November 20, 2021. https://ncsacw.acf.hhs.gov/userfiles/files/SAMHSA_Trauma.pdf
16. Barret JE. Trauma-informed nursing care. In: Gerber MR, editor. Trauma-informed healthcare approaches. Cham (Switzerland): Springer; 2019. p. 181–93.
17. Currier JM, Stefurak T, Carroll TD, et al. Applying trauma-informed care to community-based mental health services for military veterans. Best Practices MentHealth 2017;13(1):47–63.
18. Phillips GA, Lincoln YS. Introducing veteran critical theory. Int J Qual Stud Educ 2017;30(7):656–8.
19. Crenshaw K. Demarginalizing the intersection of race and sex: a black feminist critique of antidiscrimination doctrine, feminist theory and antiracist politics. Univ Chicago Leg Forum 1989;(1):139–67.
20. Testa RJ, Habarth J, Peta J, et al. Development of the gender minority stress and resilience measure. Psychol Sex Orientation Gend Divers 2015;2(1):65–77.
21. Department of Veterans Affairs National Center for Veterans Analysis and Statistics. Minority Veterans Report. 2017. Available at: https://www.va.gov/vetdata/docs/SpecialReports/Minority_Veterans_Report.pdf. Accessed December 31, 2021.
22. Levahot K, Beckman KL, Chen JA, et al. Race/ethnicity and sexual orientation disparities in mental health, sexism, and social support among women veterans. Psychol Sex Orientation Gend Divers 2019;6(3):347–58.
23. Balsam K. Trauma, stress, and resilience among sexual minority women: Rising like the phoenix. Journal of Lesbian Studies 2003;7(4):1–8.
24. Koo KH, Madden E, Maguen S. Race-ethnicity and gender differences in VA healthcare service utilization among U.S. veterans of recent conflicts. Psychiatr Serv 2016;66:507–13.

25. Chen JA, Glass JE, Bensley KMK, et al. Racial/ethnic gender differences in receipt of brief intervention among patients with unhealthy alcohol use in the U.S. Veterans Health Administration. J Substance Abuse Treat 2020;119:108078.
26. Davis DLF, DoQuyen T, Imbert E, et al. Start the way you want to finish: an intensive diversity, equity, inclusion orientation curriculum in undergraduate medical education. J Med EducCurriuculumDev 2021;8:1–6.
27. Steele C. A threat in the air: how stereotypes shape intellectual identity and performance. Am Psychol 1997;52:613–29.
28. Di Leone BAL, Wang JM, Kressin N, et al. Women's veteran identity and utilization of VA health services. Psychol Serv 2016;13(1):60–8.
29. Braun LA, Kennedy HP, Sadler LS, et al. Research on U.S. military women: recruitment and retention challenges and strategies. Mil Med 2015;180(12): 1247–55.
30. Congressional Research Service. Veterans Health Administration. 2021. Available at: https://www.everycrsreport.com/files/2021-03-11_IF11082_91bf1a09be6654cef765bbb08466f28ac48f5211.pdf. Accessed December 30, 2021.
31. Vogt D, Bergeron A, Salgado D, et al. Barriers to Veterans Health Administration care in a nationally representative sample of women veterans. J Gen Intern Med 2006;21(Suppl 3):S19–25.
32. Mattocks KM, Yano EM, Brown A, et al. Examining women veteran's experiences, perceptions, and challenges with the veterans choice program. Med Care 2018; 56(7):557–60.
33. Shipherd JC, Darling JE, Klap RS, et al. Experiences in the Veterans Health Administration and impact on healthcare utilization: comparisons between LGBT and non-LGBT women veterans. LGBT Health 2018;5(5):303–11.
34. U.S. Department of Defense. DoD instruction 1300.28: in-service transition for transgender service members. 2016. Available at: https://dod.defense.gov/Portals/1/features/2016/0616_policy/DoD-Instruction-1300.28.pdf. Accessed December 30, 2021.
35. Marchand WR, Beckstrom J, Nazarenko E, et al. The Veterans Health Administration whole health model of care: early implementation and utilization at a large healthcare system. Mil Med 2020;185(11–12):e2150–7.
36. U.S. Department of Veterans Affairs. Center for women veterans: VA women's health transition training. Available at: https://www.va.gov/womenvet/whtt/. Accessed December 29, 2021.
37. U.S. Department of Veterans Affairs. Whole Health. Available at: https://www.va.gov/wholehealth/. Accessed December 29, 2021.
38. U.S. Department of Veterans Affairs. Women Veterans Health Care. Create Community. Connect with Other Veterans. Available at: https://www.womenshealth.va.gov/WOMENSHEALTH/connect-with-other-veterans.asp. Accessed December 30, 2021.
39. National Association of State Women Veteran Coordinators. National State Women Veteran Coordinators. Available at: https://www.naswvc.org/state-coordinators-1/georgia. Accessed December 30, 2021.
40. Women Veterans Network. Available at: https://www.wovenwomenvets.org/. Accessed December 30, 2021.
41. Liu KA, Mager NA. Women's involvement in clinical trials: Historical perspective and future implications. Pharm Pract(Granada) 2016;14(1):708.
42. Danan ER, Krebs EE, Ensrud K, et al. An evidence map of the women veterans' health research literature (2008-2015). J Gen Intern Med 2017;32(12):1359–76.

43. U.S. Department of Veterans Affairs. Office of research and development. Million veteran program. Available at: https://www.research.va.gov/mvp/. Accessed December 30, 2021.
44. U.S. Department of Veterans Affairs. Million veteran program. Women veterans in research. Available at: https://www.research.va.gov/pubs/docs/va_factsheets/MVP_womens_factsheet.pdf. Accessed December 30, 2021.
45. U.S. Department of Health and Human Services. National Institutes of Health: all of us Research program. Diversity and inclusion. Available at: https://allofus.nih.gov/about. Accessed December 30, 2021.
46. Goldzweig CL, Balekian TM, Rolon C, et al. The state of women veterans' health research: results of a systematic literature review. J Gen Intern Med 2006; 21(Suppl 3):S82–92.
47. Asquith A, Sava L, Harris AB, et al. Patient-centered practices for engaging transgender and gender diverse patients in clinical research studies. BMC Med Res Methodol 2021;21(1):202.
48. U.S. Food and Drug Administration. Women in clinical trials. Available at: https://www.fda.gov/consumers/womens-health-topics/women-clinical-trials. Accessed December 30, 2021.
49. National Institutes of Health. Office of Research on Women's Health.E-Learning. Available at: https://orwh.od.nih.gov/career-development-education/e-learning. Accessed December 30, 2021.

US Department of Veterans Affairs Post-Baccalaureate Registered Nurse Residency: Developing Nurses Equipped with Knowledge and Skills to Care for Nation's Veterans

Jemma Ayvazian, DNP, ANP-BC, AOCNP, PMGT-BC, FAANP, FAAN[a,*], Beverly Gonzalez, PhD[b], Mary E. Desmond, PhD, RN, AHN-BC[b,c], Rosie Jones, MS[a], Lisa Burkhart, PhD, RN, ANEF[b,d]

KEYWORDS

• Nurse residency • New graduate nurse • Nurse competency • Veteran-centric care • Veterans

KEY POINTS

- The Veterans Affairs (VA) Office of Academic Affiliations (OAA) postbaccalaureate registered nurse residency (PB-RNR) program is designed to produce a pipeline of highly qualified, veteran health care specialty-trained registered nurses (RNs) to deliver quality care to veterans within the VA or in the community.
- The OAA-sponsored 12-month PB-RNR program provides new graduate RNs with 100% protected training time as they transition from academia to practice and develop into competent, confident nurses equipped with the knowledge and skills to care for our nation's veterans.
- PB-RNR program demonstrates effectiveness in improving new graduate nurse competence, confidence, recruitment, and retention rates in participating VA medical facilities.

[a] Office of Academic Affiliations, US Department of Veterans Affairs, 810 Vermont Avenue NW, Washington, DC 20420, USA; [b] Center of Innovation for Complex Chronic Health care, Edward Hines, Jr. VA Hospital, US Department of Veteran Affairs, 5000 5th Avenue, Hines, IL 60141, USA; [c] Master's Entry to Nursing Practice Program, DePaul University, 1 E Jackson Boulevard, Chicago, IL 60604, USA; [d] Marcella Niehoff School of Nursing, Loyola University Chicago, 1032 W Sheridan Road, Chicago, IL 60601, USA
* Corresponding author.
E-mail address: jemma.ayvazian@va.gov

Nurs Clin N Am 57 (2022) 375–392
https://doi.org/10.1016/j.cnur.2022.04.005
0029-6465/22/Published by Elsevier Inc.

Abbreviations	
VA	Department of Veterans Affairs
OAA	Office of Academic Affiliations
PB-RNR	Postbaccalaureate Registered Nurse Residency
CCNE	Commission on Collegiate Nursing Education
AY	Academic Year
RN	Registered Nurse
EBP	Evidence-Based Practice
SME	Subject Matter Expert
SA	Self-Assessment
FA	Faculty Assessment
SAS	Statistical Analysis System
COVID-19	Coronavirus Disease 2019
SD	Standard deviation
I-CVI	Item Content Validity Index

INTRODUCTION

Due to the national shortage of experienced nurses, exacerbated by pandemic-related resignations, health care organizations relied on filling nursing vacancies with new graduates or travel nurses to address the immediate staffing needs.[1] An adequate staffing by numbers only does not guarantee optimal patient care and outcomes delivery. Evidence demonstrates that an effective match between patient health care needs and nurses' knowledge, skills, and abilities is critical in delivering quality and safe patient-centered care.[2] Unfortunately, new graduate nurses face significant challenges during the transition from academia to professional clinical practice, with some expressing a lack of preparedness for practice.[3] Approximately 30% of new graduate nurses quit their job within the first 3 months of clinical practice and approximately 57% in the second year of employment.[4,5] Unsupportive work environments, fear, anxiety, and disconnect between knowledge gained in an academic program and application of skills in practice lead to "transition shock,"[3] subsequent burnout, and attrition.[4] The costs of turnover and recruitment of new nurses are high and have a profound financial and other negative impacts on health care organizations.[6,7] Average-sized hospitals lose $7.1 million due to registered nurse (RN) turnover costs each year.[6] The literature suggests that implementing and managing a structured nurse residency program can increase the supply of skilled nurses by improving nurse competence, confidence in practice, and retention, whilereducing recruitment and turnover costs.

Since 2002, several national organizations, including the Joint Commission, the National Academy of Medicine, the National Council of State Boards of Nursing, and the Commission on Collegiate Nursing Education (CCNE), advocated for the establishment of nurse residency programs to support nurse graduates transition from academia to clinical practice.[5,8] The implementation and evaluation of effective nurse residency programs are multifaceted and complex. When designing a nurse residency program, it is critical to align program theoretic grounding with the outcome and process goals that are measured with theoretically, conceptually consistent, and psychometrically supported instruments. Despite the abundance of nurse residency literature, there are gaps identified by the lack of psychometrically sound program evaluation tools[9] and outcomes related to population-specific specialty knowledge, skills, and competency development.[10]

Military and veteran populations have unique health concerns related to specific service histories,[11] which require specialized knowledge and skills.[12] Veterans have higher rates of psychosocial conditions, including depression, posttraumatic stress disorder, substance abuse disorder, suicide, and homelessness.[12] Specific military experiences also introduce physical disorders, including traumatic brain injury, chronic pain, amputations, spinal cord injury, and hazardous exposures associated with particular deployment and tours of duty (e.g., agent orange, burn pit smoke).[12]

The veteran population is growing, with many veterans receiving care outside of the Veterans Affairs (VA) health care system. In 2017, only half of veterans (9.8 million out of 20.0 million) used at least one VA benefit or service, including health care, compensation or pension, life insurance, education, memorial benefits, vocational rehabilitation, and housing benefits.[13] From 2008 to 2017, there was a significant growth in the utilization of VA health care services by veterans. In 2017, VA health care services were used by one-third of the total veteran population (6.1 million veterans).[13] The likelihood of veterans seeking VA health care increases with the service-connected disability rating (overall utilization rate among disabled veterans is 69.6%).[13] Nonetheless, the data indicated that a large proportion of the veteran population received health care in the community. In addition, under the VA Mission Act of 2018 (Public Law 115–182),[14] veterans who receive VA health care are eligible and may choose to receive certain services from community providers.

These trends require academia and the VA to work together to ensure that all health care providers possess the required knowledge and skills to provide quality care to our nation's veterans. Unfortunately, nursing education programs have not traditionally incorporated military and veteran-specific content in RN prelicensure curricula, leaving a gap in new graduate nurses' knowledge and skills related to care for veterans. The lack of military and veteran-specific health care competency affects the ability of new graduate nurses hired by the VA to promptly assimilate into the VA health care environment and provide effective services to the veteran population. Moreover, the nursing workforce that had never trained or worked within the VA health care system frequently lacks the veteran-specific health care knowledge required to address the specific needs of this population. The purpose of this article is to discuss the VA Office of Academic Affiliations (OAA) postbaccalaureate registered nurse residency (PB-RNR) model and its effectiveness in developing confident new graduate RNs equipped with the knowledge and skills to care for our nation's veterans within the VA and the community.

Veterans Affairs Office of Academic Affiliations Postbaccalaureate Registered Nurse Residency Program

The PB-RNR program is designed to produce a pipeline of highly qualified, veteran health care specialty-trained RNs (bachelor's, master's, or doctoral prepared RNs) to deliver quality care to veterans within the VA or community. Since 2011, the OAA has piloted several nurse residency models to identify successful strategies. The pilot programs provided a platform and structure for successfully launching the VA Nurse Residency Expansion Initiative in 2018. Currently, OAA funds 49 PB-RNR programs.

The PB-RNR programs were approved at selected VA medical facilities through a Requests for Proposals process and underwent a rigorous three-step review process. Each proposal was assigned a primary, secondary, and tertiary subject matter expert (SME) reviewer, often an experienced PB-RNR program director at an existing site. Step 1 included individual SME reviews to assess and rate the submitted proposal against the established objective rubric. In addition, the OAA held a 2-hour training session with reviewers before each review process to achieve high interrater reliability.

Step 2 included a review panel teleconference, during which reviewers presented their findings, discussed the strengths and weaknesses of each proposal, and reached a consensus on a recommendation for funding. Step 3 consisted of a review of recommendations for funding by OAA senior leaders and approval or disapproval of the proposal.

The PB-RNR program is a year-long, competency-based training delivered in collaboration with a school of nursing. To enter the PB-RNR, residents must be licensed RNs, serving in their first RN role and having graduated within the previous 12 months from a baccalaureate, master's, or doctoral level course of study accredited by the CCNE or the Accreditation Commission for Education in Nursing. The OAAs RN residents are appointed as VA trainees, do not have a service-obligation requirement at the completion of residency, and may choose to stay at the VA or seek employment in the private sector after graduation.

Each PB-RNR program has a veteran-centric curriculum with defined didactic and experiential learning activities focused on advancing clinical, leadership, interprofessional, scholarship skills, and military/veteran-centric care knowledge and culture. Most of the didactic training is centered on learning about the military and veteran culture and expanding a health care knowledge base. The OAA's competency-based RN residency curriculum is based on an 80/20 model with 80% of training time spent in hands-on training and 20% in didactics. The curriculum is aligned with CCNE accreditation standards and VA RN competency requirements. The curriculum model is designed to allow new graduate nurses to apply knowledge and skills gained during prelicensure educational experiences across various VA clinical settings to advance their skills.

The PB-RNR residents have 100% protected training time during their 12 months of training at the VA medical facility to master the complexities of caring for veterans. Residents practice under the supervision of experienced VA RN clinical faculty/preceptors and, in addition to their primary assignment unit, complete multiple rotations of various complexity and acuity of care during the year-long training. Clinical training is structured to gradually increase the complexity of assignments and progression from lower to higher acuities of care delivery. The combination of robust didactic and clinical experiences coupled with protected training time for the entire duration of the PB-RNR program allows new graduate RNs to focus on the identification of strengths and weaknesses, enhancement of competencies, and engagement in professional development, distinguishing the OAA nurse residency from employee-based on-the-job training models.

Evidence-based practice (EBP) is a central tenet of the residency program. During the year-long training at VA medical facilities, PB-RNR residents are required to complete a quality enhancement or system redesign scholarly project focused on improving the quality, access, and cost of health care. PB-RNR residents may choose to conduct individual or group scholarly projects, depending on the facility's individual needs and residents' skills. It is strongly advised that EBP projects be identified and established in collaboration with VA medical facility executive leaders to ensure the economical, technical, and operational feasibility of the project to address that facility's immediate needs.

Each PB-RNR training site has a dedicated program director responsible for designing, implementing, and managing the program based on the local VA medical facility needs with ongoing support from the OAA. The VA headquarters centrally funds PB-RNR trainee positions, paying the stipends and benefits, and reimburses the salary of the VA medical facility PB-RNR program director to ensure dedicated administrative time for program management. All PB-RNR programs have a requirement to obtain accreditation by the CCNE within 3 years of implementation.

METHODS

The OAA developed and implemented an extensive, multidimensional, program-specific national evaluation plan to monitor the effectiveness of its programs. The evaluation is built on a mixed-methods approach with four intended goals: (1) improve the new graduate RNs' overall competency and confidence in practice within the VA health care setting; (2) improve new graduate RNs' knowledge and skills related to veteran care; (3) enhance VA recruitment and retention of new graduate RNs; and (4) identify challenges and recommendations for ongoing program improvement. The PB-RNR program data collection occurred via an electronic data portal developed and maintained by the OAA. The data were collected at predetermined intervals. The appropriate analytical method for evaluating each aim was determined based on the data type and variables of interest. Quantitative statistical analyses were conducted via statistical analysis system (SAS) software, version 9.4 (SAS Institute Inc, 2013), R Core Team (2013), and Microsoft Excel. In addition, qualitative data analyses were conducted by two experienced qualitative researchers using tables in Microsoft Word.

Instrumentation

Postbaccalaureate registered nurse residency competency assessment

The OAA PB-RNR Competency Assessment Instrument is an RN skills competency instrument developed to evaluate individual RN resident performance in 22 core clinical competency areas organized into 11 domains consistent with CCNE RN Residency Accreditation Standards and the VA veteran-centric model of care (**Table 1**). The instrument has two components: (1) Resident Competency Self-Assessment and (2) Faculty-rated Competency Assessment of resident's performance. The Resident Competency Self-Assessment is completed by each PB-RNR resident at program entry (1 month) and program completion (12 months) to measure self-perceived competency in clinical skills. The Faculty-rated Competency Assessment of residents' performance was conducted at predetermined intervals: program entry (1 month), interim (3 months and 6 months), and completion of the program (12 months).

Tool refinement and content validity were evaluated by experts from both academic and clinical service settings using the I-CVI method (scored on a 4-point Likert scale, strongly disagree to strongly agree) with four expert RNs from both academic and clinical service settings, reaching 100% agreement (agree or strongly agree) after two rounds. The resulting tool measures each competency based on the performance criteria of 1 to 12 items. The instrument rating scale is built on Benner's Novice to Expert model[15] and the Entrustment of Professional Activities,[16,17] which is based on the level of supervision needed to carry out the activity. The skill levels are defined as follows: 1 = resident demonstrates critical deficiencies in knowledge, skills, and attitude to safely perform the task; 2 = resident performs the task under the direct guidance of faculty (greater than 75% of the time); 3 = resident performs the task under extensive guidance of the faculty (50%–75% of the time); 4 = resident performs the task under frequent guidance of faculty (25%–50% of the time); 5 = resident performs the task under occasional guidance of the faculty (less than 25% of the time); and 6 = resident performs the task safely and effectively using own judgment without supporting cues. We tested (via R Core Team [2013] polychoric function) the scale

Table 1
Comparison of faculty and postbaccalaureate nurse residency self-assessments ordinal Cronbach's alpha by domains and competency at baseline (1 month) and completion (12 months)

	Cronbach's Alpha			
	Baseline		Completion	
Domain/Competency Category	SA	FA	SA	FA
DOMAIN: QUALITY/SAFETY	0.98	0.99	0.99	0.99
COMP 1. Culture of patient safety	0.96	0.96	0.96	0.97
COMP 2. Fall prevention	0.97	0.98	0.97	0.99
COMP 3. Infection control and prevention	0.95	0.96	0.99	0.96
COMP 4. Medication administration	0.97	0.97	0.96	0.97
COMP 5. Evidence-based skin care practice	0.97	0.97	0.97	0.98
DOMAIN: PATIENT AND FAMILY CENTERED CARE	0.99	0.99	0.99	0.99
COMP 6. Patient/family education	0.97	0.98	0.97	0.98
COMP 7. Assessment and management of pain	0.97	0.97	0.97	0.98
COMP 8. End of life care	0.97	0.97	0.96	0.98
COMP 9. Military and veteran-centric care	0.98	0.98	0.98	0.99
COMP 10. Cultural competency	0.98	0.98	1.00	0.99
DOMAIN: MANAGEMENT OF PATIENT CARE DELIVERY	0.98	0.98	0.99	0.99
COMP 11. Management of patient care delivery	0.98	0.99	0.99	0.99
COMP 12. Interprofessional collaboration	0.95	0.95	0.99	0.97
COMP 13. Resource management	0.96	9.96	0.97	0.97
DOMAIN: MANAGEMENT OF THE CHANGING PATIENT CONDITION	0.98	0.98	0.98	0.99
COMP 14. Management of the changing patient condition	0.98	0.98	0.98	0.99
DOMAIN: COMMUNICATION AND CONFLICT MANAGEMENT	0.97	0.98	0.98	0.98
COMP 15. Communication	0.95	0.96	0.98	0.88
COMP 16. Conflict management	0.96	0.96	0.97	0.98
DOMAIN: INFORMATICS AND TECHNOLOGY	0.95	0.96	0.98	0.97
COMP 17. Informatics and technology	0.95	0.96	0.98	0.97
DOMAIN: PROFESSIONAL DEVELOPMENT	0.94	0.96	0.96	0.97
COMP 18. Professional development	0.94	0.96	0.96	0.97
DOMAIN: EVIDENCE-BASED PRACTICE	0.97	0.98	0.97	0.99
COMP 19. Evidence-based practice	0.97	0.98	0.97	0.99
DOMAIN: ETHICAL DECISION-MAKING	0.94	0.94	0.97	0.97
COMP 20. Ethical decision-making	0.94	0.94	0.97	0.97
DOMAIN: STRESS management	0.96	0.99	0.95	0.97
COMP 21. Stress management	0.96	0.99	0.95	0.97
DOMAIN: BUSINESS OF HEALTH CARE	0.95	0.96	0.94	0.97
COMP 22. Business of health care	0.95	0.96	0.94	0.97

Abbreviations: FA, faculty assessment; SA, PBRNR resident self-assessment.

reliability of the PB-RNR competency instrument by generating Cronbach's alpha used for ordinal scales as a measure of internal consistency for competencies and domains, with alpha scores >0.9 (see **Table 1**).

Postbaccalaureate registered nurse residency confidence in practice

PB-RNR confidence in practice was measured using the Casey-Fink Graduate Nurse Experience Survey.[18] The Confidence in Practice Survey was designed to evaluate the residents' comfort and confidence in their transition to the role of a professional nurse as it pertains to the performance of core clinical skills and abilities. The survey includes five subscales: communication and leadership, organizing and prioritizing, professional satisfaction, stress, and support. PB-RNR residents completed the confidence survey: at program entry (1 month), interim (3 months and 6 months), and completion of the program (12 months).

Postbaccalaureate registered nurse residency program annual report

The PB-RNR program annual report is designed to collect program outcome data related to the successful implementation of the year-long VA postbaccalaureate residency. The report is completed annually by the PB-RNR program director at individual training sites within 30 days of residency graduation. Key elements include resident enrollment, recruitment, and retention data; program faculty data; program accreditation status; the number and type (quality, access, or cost) of scholarly projects completed by residents; and challenges, lessons learned, and recommendations for ongoing program improvement.

Analyses

To test whether resident self-assessment (SA) and faculty assessment (FA) in mean rating competency scores changed over the 12-month program, we invoked repeated measures (also known as within-group design) in which the same residents took part at each interval entry (1 month, 3 months, 6 months, and 12 months). We denote these interval entry values in the analysis within a timepoint variable (having values of either 1, 3, 6, or 12). In addition, the resident confidence in practice was assessed similarly using generalized models rating confidence score changes for each PB-RNR SA timepoint. Hence, our null and alternative hypotheses at a two-tailed significance level of 0.05 were as follows:

H_0: There is no change in mean competency (SA and FA) and confidence in practice (SA) rating scores over the 12-month program.

H_1: The mean change in competency (SA and FA) and confidence in practice (SA) rating scores over the 12-month program was not equal to 0.

Program directors reported the number and type of EBP projects completed through a web-based annual report. The number and type of projects were tabulated and summarized. Over the 5 years of program implementation, PB-RNR program directors submitted qualitative data via the annual report describing challenges and lessons learned related to trainee selection, recruitment, retention, and program implementation. Program directors also identified recommendations and critical support. Two experienced qualitative researchers analyzed narrative data using content analysis.[19]

Program start dates were staggered throughout the academic year (AY): 14 in 2016, with 3 additional dates in 2018 and 8 additional dates in 2020. To evaluate change over time, data were sorted and analyzed by program implementation year (beginning with start year) in chronological order rather than actual academic year order. That is, all

Table 2
Characteristics of study population

PB-NRN Characteristic	n (%)
Age mean (SD) (years)	27 (8.11)
Sex	
Female	330 (76.57%)
Male	101 (23.43%)
Race	
White	268 (62.18%)
Black	49 (11.37%)
Hispanic	57 (13.23%)
Indian	2 (0.46%)
Asian	45 (10.44%)
Asian/Pacific Islander	4 (0.93%)
Other	6 (1.39%)
Highest degree earned	
BSN	424 (98.38%)
MSN	5 (1.16%)
Prior work experience	
Nursing assistant	141 (32.71%)
Student nurse technician	57 (13.23%)
Nurse extern	29 (6.73%)
VALOR student program	34 (7.89%)
Military corpsman/medic	16 (3.71%)
Emergency medical technician	13 (3.02%)
Military service	63 (14.62%)
Total population	431

programs reported data for the first year of implementation regardless of what calendar year the program began or how long the program existed. This approach allowed identifying trends based on experience in implementing the program. Each qualitative researcher individually analyzed responses to each question using open coding to identify key categories, followed by a discussion to refine and define the categories, beginning with the first program year and then sequentially to 5 years. Data saturated at the categorical level over the course of the 5 years.

RESULTS

In AY 2017, AY 2018, AYo 2019, and AY 2020, the number of RN residents who participated in the PB-RNR program and completed all assessments at all timepoints varied. A total of 431 trainees completed both SA and FA at all time points. The baseline characteristics of the study population are presented in **Table 2**. The mean age of the study population was 27 years. Most of the residents were women (76.57%). Most of the residents were White (62.18%), followed by Hispanic (13.23%), Black (11.37%), and Asian (10.44%). Most residents had a Bachelor of Science in Nursing (BSN) degree (98.38%), whereas a small percentage (1.16%) had a Master of Science in Nursing (MSN) degree. This cohort also indicated some prior

Table 3
Differences of least-squares means for postbaccalaureate nurse residency competencies

Competency	LS means at each timepoint (FA)					LS means at each timepoint (SA)		
	Month 1 Estimate (SE)	Month 3 Estimate (SE	Month 1 Estimate (SE)	Month 12 Estimate (SE)	1–12 month Change (SE)[a]	Month 1 Estimate (SE)	Month 12 Estimate (SE)	1–12 month Change (SE)[a]
COMP 1. Culture of patient safety	3.52 (0.05)	4.08 (0.04)	3.32 (0.05)	5.44 (0.03)	2.12 (0.05)[a]	4.61 (0.04)	5.48 (0.03)	1.96 (0.05)[a]
COMP 2. Fall prevention	3.78 (0.05)	4.41 (0.05)	3.64 (0.05)	5.72 (0.03)	2.08 (0.05)[a]	4.99 (0.04)	5.68 (0.03)	1.90 (0.05)[a]
COMP 3. Infection control and prevention	3.69 (0.05)	4.31 (0.04)	3.54 (0.04)	5.60 (0.02)	2.06 (0.05)[a]	4.86 (0.04)	5.57 (0.03)	1.88 (0.05)[a]
COMP 4. Medication administration	3.43 (0.04)	4.14 (0.04)	3.28 (0.05)	5.51 (0.03)	2.23 (0.05)[a]	4.70 (0.04)	5.47 (0.03)	2.04 (0.05)[a]
COMP 5. Evidence-based skin care practice	3.55 (0.05)	4.27 (0.04)	3.46 (0.04)	5.64 (0.03)	2.18 (0.05)[a]	4.83 (0.03)	5.59 (0.03)	2.04 (0.05)[a]
COMP 6. Patient/family education	3.28 (0.04)	4.07 (0.04)	3.27 (0.05)	5.55 (0.03)	2.28 (0.05)[a]	4.63 (0.04)	5.48 (0.03)	2.10 (0.05)[a]
COMP 7. Assessment and management of pain	3.54 (0.05)	4.24 (0.04)	3.50 (0.05)	5.63 (0.03)	2.13 (0.05)[a]	4.82 (0.04)	5.60 (0.03)	2.06 (0.05)[a]
COMP 8. End of life care	2.99 (0.05)	3.59 (0.05)	3.03 (0.05)	5.23 (0.04)	2.20 (0.06)[a]	4.17 (0.04)	5.11 (0.04)	2.11 (0.06)[a]
COMP 9. Military and veteran-centric care	2.94 (0.04)	3.54 (0.04)	2.91 (0.04)	5.19 (0.04)	2.27 (0.05)[a]	4.07 (0.04)	5.00 (0.04)	2.07 (0.05)[a]
COMP 10. Cultural competency	3.82 (0.05)	4.45 (0.05)	3.84 (0.05)	5.73 (0.03)	1.89 (0.06)[a]	5.02 (0.04)	5.66 (0.03)	1.85 (0.06)[a]
COMP 11. Management of patient care delivery	3.24 (0.04)	4.01 (0.04)	3.19 (0.04)	5.59 (0.03)	2.40 (0.05)[a]	4.63 (0.04)	5.48 (0.03)	2.24 (0.05)[a]
COMP 12. Interprofessional collaboration	3.95 (0.05)	4.53 (0.05)	3.94 (0.05)	5.78 (0.03)	1.84 (0.05)[a]	5.05 (0.04)	5.72 (0.03)	1.76 (0.05)[a]
COMP 13. Resource management	3.47 (0.05)	4.13 (0.05)	3.41 (0.05)	5.62 (0.03)	2.22 (0.06)[a]	4.79 (0.04)	5.51 (0.03)	2.05 (0.06)[a]
COMP 14. Management of the changing patient condition	3.32 (0.05)	4.07 (0.04)	3.27 (0.05)	5.59 (0.03)	2.32 (0.05)[a]	4.66 (0.04)	5.51 (0.03)	2.19 (0.05)[a]
COMP 15. Communication	3.71 (0.05)	4.42 (0.04)	3.58 (0.05)	5.73 (0.03)	2.16 (0.05)[a]	5.01 (0.04)	5.68 (0.03)	1.97 (0.05)[a]
COMP 16. Conflict management	3.44 (0.05)	4.09 (0.04)	3.53 (0.05)	5.57 (0.03)	2.03 (0.06)[a]	4.69 (0.04)	5.48 (0.03)	2.03 (0.06)[a]
COMP 17. Informatics and technology	3.59 (0.05)	4.33 (0.04)	3.49 (0.05)	5.69 (0.03)	2.20 (0.06)[a]	4.93 (0.04)	5.63 (0.03)	2.04 (0.06)[a]
COMP 18. Professional development	3.74 (0.05)	4.38 (0.05)	3.79 (0.05)	5.71 (0.03)	1.92 (0.06)[a]	4.90 (0.04)	5.61 (0.03)	1.87 (0.06)[a]
COMP 19. Evidence-based practice	3.21 (0.04)	3.85 (0.05)	3.15 (0.04)	5.47 (0.03)	2.31 (0.05)[a]	4.44 (0.04)	5.31 (0.03)	2.10 (0.05)[a]

(continued on next page)

Table 3
(continued)

Competency	LS means at each timepoint (FA)					LS means at each timepoint (SA)		
	Month 1 Estimate (SE)	Month 3 Estimate (SE	Month 1 Estimate (SE)	Month 12 Estimate (SE)	1–12 month Change (SE)[a]	Month 1 Estimate (SE)	Month 12 Estimate (SE)	1–12 month Change (SE)[a]
COMP 20. Ethical decision-making	3.71 (0.05)	4.38 (0.05)	3.83 (0.05)	5.71 (0.03)	1.88 (0.06)[a]	4.97 (0.04)	5.63 (0.03)	1.92 (0.06)[a]
COMP 21. Stress management	3.76 (0.05)	4.38 (0.05)	3.80 (0.05)	5.65 (0.03)	1.85 (0.06)[a]	4.91 (0.04)	5.58 (0.03)	1.82 (0.06)[a]
COMP 22. Business of health care	3.16 (0.05)	3.89 (0.05)	3.11 (0.05)	5.41 (0.04)	2.30 (0.05)[a]	4.44 (0.04)	5.34 (0.04)	2.18 (0.05)[a]

Abbreviations: FA, faculty assessment; LS, least-squares means; SA, PBRNR resident self-assessment; SE, standard error.

[a] $p < .0001$ for all competencies.

Table 4
Differences of least-squares means for military and veteran-centric care competency

	LS Means at Each Timepoint (FA)					LS Means at Each Timepoint (SA)		
Competency Item	**Month 1 Estimate (SE)**	**Month 3 Estimate (SE)**	**Month 6 Estimate (SE)**	**Month 12 Estimate (SE)**	**1–12 month Change (SE)[a]**	**Month 1 Estimate (SE)**	**Month 12 Estimate (SE)**	**1–12 month Change (SE)[a]**
Agent orange exposure-related diseases	2.67 (0.04)	3.29 (0.04)	3.84 (0.05	4.79 (0.04)	2.12 (0.06)[a]	2.51 (0.04)	5.01 (0.04)	2.50 (0.06)[a]
Combat-related mental health	3.17 (0.05)	3.80 (0.05)	4.37 (0.05)	5.25 (0.04)	2.08 (0.06)[a]	3.19 (0.05)	5.48 (0.04)	2.28 (0.06)[a]
Deployment-related immunizations	2.69 (0.05)	3.24 (0.05)	3.78 (0.05)	4.70 (0.05)	2.00 (0.07)[a]	2.62 (0.05)	4.88 (0.05)	2.26 (0.07)[a]
Substance use disorders in military/vet population	3.17 (0.05)	3.81 (0.05)	4.32 (0.05)	5.25 (0.04)	2.08 (0.06)[a]	3.18 (0.05)	5.50 (0.04)	2.32 (0.06)[a]
Military sexual trauma	2.84 (0.05)	3.41(0.05)	3.96 (0.05)	4.91 (0.05)	2.07 (0.06)[a]	2.77 (0.05)	5.12 (0.05)	2.34 (0.06)[a]
Traumatic brain injury	2.95 (0.05)	3.57 (0.05)	4.09 (0.05)	5.03 (0.04)	2.08 (0.06)[a]	2.99 (0.05)	5.20 (0.04)	2.22 (0.06)[a]
Burn injuries	2.76 (0.05)	3.27 (0.05)	3.71 (0.05)	4.74 (0.05)	1.97 (0.07)[a]	2.83 (0.05)	4.77 (0.05)	1.94 (0.07)[a]
Spinal cord injuries	2.89 (0.05)	3.46 (0.05)	3.97 (0.05)	4.89 (0.05)	1.99 (0.06)[a]	2.91 (0.05)	5.05 (0.05)	2.13 (0.06)[a]
Amputation/assistive devices	2.98 (0.05)	3.67 (0.05)	4.24 (0.05)	5.17 (0.04)	2.19 (0.06)[a]	2.97 (0.05)	5.34 (0.04)	2.37 (0.06)[a]
Veteran women health issues	2.88 (0.05)	3.46 (0.05)	3.98 (0.05)	4.90 (0.05)	2.03 (0.06)[a]	2.70 (0.05)	5.07 (0.05)	2.37 (0.06)[a]
Homelessness/socioeconomic concerns	3.10 (0.05)	3.76 (0.05)	4.25 (0.05)	5.19 (0.04)	2.09 (0.06)[a]	3.10 (0.05)	5.40 (0.04)	2.29 (0.06)[a]
Suicide	3.12 (0.05)	3.73 (0.05)	4.28 (0.05)	5.23 (0.04)	2.11 (0.06)[a]	3.20 (0.05)	5.40 (0.04)	2.21 (0.06)[a]

Abbreviations: FA, faculty assessment; LS, least-squares means; SA, PBRNR resident self-assessment; SE, standard error.
[a] $p < .0001$ for all competencies.

nursing work experience: Nursing Assistant (32.71%), Student Nurse Technician (13.23%), Nurse Extern (6.73%), VA Learning Opportunities Residency (VALOR) Nurse Student (7.89%), Military Corpsman/Medic (3.71%), and Emergency Medical Technician (3.02%). Approximately 14.62% served in the military.

Postbaccalaureate Registered Nurse Residency Competency Assessment

Over the 12-month program, for all 22 competencies and all data sets analyzed, the least-squares means (lsmeans) rating score changes (for each of SA and FA) were consistently highly statistically significant ($p < .0001$), as shown in **Table 3**. The lsmeans is a linear combination of the parameter estimates in the model that are known as adjusted means. In addition, for FA, the other pairs of timepoint comparisons (1–3, 3–6, 6–12) were also statistically significant ($p < .05$), with timepoint comparisons (1–12) that were generally highly statistically significant ($p < .0001$).

Military and Veteran-Centric Care Knowledge

For all 12 items under veteran-centric competency, the lsmeans rating score changes over the 12-month program were highly statistically significant ($p < .0001$) for both SA and FA (**Table 4**). For FA, the other pairs of timepoint comparisons (1–3, 3–6, and 6–12) were also all statistically significant and generally highly statistically significant ($p < .0001$).

Postbaccalaureate Registered Nurse Residency Confidence in Practice

Over the 12-month program, the change in resident confidence statistically significantly increased ($p < .0001$) overall and for each subscale except for stress, as shown in **Fig. 1**.

Postbaccalaureate Registered Nurse Residency Veterans Affairs Recruitment and Retention

Recruitment and retention data used for analyses were self-reported by the VA medical facilities. In addition, the VA recruitment (i.e., hired by VA post-residency) data

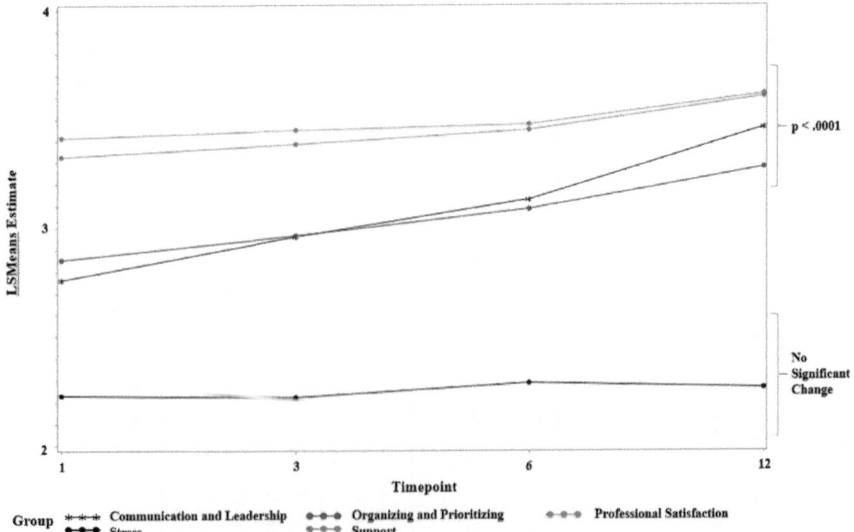

Fig. 1. Progression of PB-RNR confidence in practice by subscales.

include the reports of hires at the local VA facilities, where the residency program was conducted, and "other" VA medical facilities (nationally). Currently, there is no mechanism to accurately track national PB-RNR program graduate recruitment data. Hence, the results presented below are based on local VA medical facility data reported by the residency program directors.

Based on data reported during academic year (AY) 2015 to 2021, the VA aggregate recruitment rate of PB-RNR graduates was 92%, indicating that VA medical facilities recruited most of the graduates. Of 739 PB-RNR graduates, 681 were hired by the VA. According to the residency program directors, reasons that graduates were not hired included graduates seeking positions in the civilian sector for desired specialty/shift not available at the VA (e.g., obstetrics on day shift), personal reasons (e.g., moving), or returning to graduate school. In addition, the 1-year VA retention rate of PB-RNR graduates was 94% based on data reported from AY 2015 to 2019. Of 390 graduates hired by VA locally, 368 remained employed by the VA 12 months posthire.

Postbaccalaureate Registered Nurse Residency Evidence-Based Projects

Over 5 years, residents completed 261 EBP projects to enhance quality, improve access, and/or decrease cost: 46 projects in 2016, 48 projects in 2017, 54 projects in 2018, 48 projects in 2019, and 65 projects in 2020. From 2016 to 2019, all participating VA medical facilities that hosted the PB-RNR program reported implementing at least one EBP project by residents. Evidence-based project outcomes reported by the program directors at individual VA medical facilities supported organizational initiatives to enhance quality, improve access, and decrease cost.

Challenges, Lessons Learned, and Recommendations

Twenty-five PB-RNR programs submitted qualitative data in the annual report, identifying program implementation challenges, lessons learned, and recommendations.

Program implementation challenges

Program implementation challenges related to program start-up included recruiting candidates, adapting the program to site differences, maintaining a supply of trained clinical faculty/preceptors, and managing COVID-19 protocols.

- Program Start-up: Each program experienced initial challenges such as engaging health systems and academic partner stakeholders, hiring program directors, developing the PB-RNR resident position, developing training program policies and procedures, and creating didactic and clinical experiences. Program directors needed support in initiating CCNE accreditation. Most of these challenges were resolved over the first few years. The VA OAA provided additional support and established the VA OAA PB-RNR National SharePoint to share resources.
- Recruitment to the Program: Recruitment of PB-RNR trainee challenges differed per site and over time, depending on the supply and demand of RNs and competition from other health systems, offering high salaries and sign-on bonuses. Marketing and collaboration with academic partners were critical to address recruitment to the program.
- Adapting the Program to Site Differences: Each site was affected by geographic differences in RN graduation dates. In addition, PB-RNR program start times did not necessarily align with RN academic program graduation and National Council Licensure Examination pass notifications. For example, nursing schools may hold graduations in spring, summer, and fall, whereas the PB-RNR program initially began in July per the VA official academic year. The VA OAA later allowed for flexibility in program start times to address these challenges.

- Maintaining a Supply of Trained Clinical Faculty/Preceptors: Maintaining a robust supply of clinical faculty/preceptors to prevent burnout was also a challenge, particularly in year 4.
- Managing COVID-19 Protocols: COVID-19 introduced challenges in education and clinical experiences. Education and simulation were moved online or canceled. Clinical rotations were modified based on institutional policy (e.g., adding telehealth, limiting rotations off home units).

Lessons learned

Strong organizational and leadership support was critical for nurse residency program success. This included a multifaceted approach in stakeholder engagement and program implementation at all levels of the health system with support from academic partners and OAA:

- Organizational senior leadership support and commitment to the program's overall goals and funding (e.g., accreditation fees, resident conference attendance, purchase of training resources and materials)
- Collaboration with academic partners to ensure the success and quality of the program (e.g., curriculum design, faculty, accreditation)
- Nurse manager support for the program (e.g., match residents with unit/experiential training, ensure preceptor protected time, monitor a reasonable workload for preceptors)
- Unit staff support of the PB-RNR residents/program (e.g., interdisciplinary team members support, recognition of RN and not student role)
- Information technology support (e.g., equipment, virtual training support)
- SME engagement in education planning (e.g., nurse educators, interprofessional education)
- Support of VA medical facility quality improvement and assurance personnel, including the EBP coordinator, to facilitate residents' EBP projects
- Training for VA medical facility nurse recruiters and human resources to onboard PB-RNR residents and VA hiring of graduates in a timely manner
- A strong, engaged, committed, competent preceptor pool on each unit to meet the program's/residents' needs and prevent preceptor burnout
- Protected time for preceptors to perform program activities (e.g., attend training sessions, complete trainee evaluations)
- Dedicated classroom space/equipment, simulation laboratory, clinical resources, computer access, and administrative office space

Recommendations

Given the multifaceted and robust nature of the PB-RNR program, establishing a strong VA-academic partnership at the individual VA medical facility level is essential for program design, implementation, and delivery (e.g., curriculum development, program evaluation, clinicalfaculty/preceptor training, program accreditation, ongoing program improvement activities). As most of the nursing predegree academic programs do not currently incorporate military and veteran health care-related content in curricula, most of the residents entering the PB-RNR program lacked basic knowledge of veteran population needs. To close the gap in PB-RNR residents' knowledge of veteran care delivery, programs are advised to front-load this didactic education content early in the PB-RNR training program. In addition, to enhance resident recruitment efforts, individual VA medical facilities are encouraged to consider flexibility with PB-RNR program start dates (spring, summer, fall) to align with academic affiliate RN program graduation dates.

DISCUSSION

The multidimensional evaluation of the PB-RNR program provides insight into the ways and methods of establishing and managing nurse residency programs in large health care organizations with multisite program delivery. Standardizing program requirements throughout the health care organization, including the program curriculum and evaluation using psychometrically supported tools, is essential in ensuring the success and effectiveness of these training programs. Our findings demonstrate that nurse residency programs, established in collaboration with academic partners, enhanced new graduate nurse competency and confidence in practice, served as an effective bridge between academia and practice for new graduate nurses, and increased VA nurse recruitment and retention of skilled nurses.

The first year of clinical practice is critical in enculturing the new graduate into professional practice and the unique aspects of veteran care. The study results demonstrate statistically significantly improved competence of new RN graduates after completion of the PB-RNR program for all 22 assessed competencies compared with baseline assessment at program entry. At the same time, the overall new graduate confidence level improved in communication, leadership, organizing, prioritizing, professional satisfaction, and support, with the highest gain occurring between 6 months and 12 months.

The PB-RNR program curriculum, in addition to experiential training, incorporated multimodal didactic education activities to include case analysis, simulation, clinical coaching, escape rooms, journaling, and journal clubs. The education content was holistic in that it incorporated knowledge and skills related to physical care (e.g., pathophysiology, skills, pharmacology, medication management, skincare, military exposures), cultural diversity, end-of-life issues, conflict management, and social issues. The evidence-based project activities provided an opportunity for PB-RNR trainees to experience teamwork, demonstrate leadership, and build confidence in supporting institutional quality, access, and cost initiatives in a continuous learning environment. Adding a flexible educational component to the residency improved needed clinical competence and confidence due to the loss of clinical predegree experiences while minimizing stress and instilling professional, institutional values in the new nurse graduates.[1] These initiatives are consistent with the National Academy of Medicine Future of Nursing Report calling for employers and schools of nursing to create a pipeline of prepared nurse leaders that support health equity and promote nurses' health and well-being.[20]

Of note, PB-RNR trainee stress levels maintained a low level over the 12-month training program, supporting the effectiveness of the residency in mitigating burnout over the first transitional year after graduation. The high recruitment and 1-year retention of RNs post-residency to full-time positions also support this success. The residency is designed to minimize the current trends of burnout and high turnover among new graduate nurses.

Health care and nursing organizations have recognized the importance of nurse self-care in both nursing education and practice.[20–23] Nurses care for patients at the moment of need, often during times of crisis. These experiences affect nurses and require reflection to find meaning and a sense of purpose.[24] Nursing caring theory, simulation, intentional debriefing, and reflective practices can help guide nurse self-care to increase resilience and prevent burnout.[20,24–27] The residency program provides an opportunity for nurses to develop reflective practices and build a supportive community to care for themselves and others.

At the baseline assessment (program entry), new nurse graduates demonstrated military and veteran care competence knowledge gaps. The PB-RNR program successfully addressed this gap, demonstrating significant improvement in veteran-centric competency on completion of the residency program. Our results support the need for a VA nurse residency to ensure that nurses are competent in addressing the unique needs of the vulnerable veteran population. In addition, the residency program required collaboration with academic partners. Academic and practice partnerships provided an opportunity to integrate veteran care competencies into predegree curricula and enhance curricula in postdegree training programs. Many veterans receive care in the civilian sector; therefore, integrating veteran care competencies in nursing schools' RN predegree curriculum is necessary to prepare nurse graduates to care for this vulnerable population within the VA and the community. The PB-RNR program provides an opportunity to further develop a bridge between academia and practice to support veteran health.

SUMMARY

The OAA's PB-RNR residents improved by self- and faculty-rating scores in competency skills and confidence in practice after the training program. In addition, the established PB-RNR competency assessment tool demonstrated a high overall internal consistency (among individual competencies and domains) when scored by residents and faculty. The PB-RNR residents supported quality improvement initiatives at VA medical facilities by completing EBP projects to improve quality, increase access, and reduce costs. High recruitment and 1-year retention rates of residency graduates result in significant organizational benefits. The evaluation results provided evidence for the effectiveness of the PB-RNR program in developing well equipped nurses to care for our nation's veterans and offered insight into areas in which improvement in the program can be made.

CLINICS CARE POINTS

- Effective nurse residency programs require strong collaboration between academia and practice.
- Nursing workforce must be equipped with the military- and veteran-specific knowledge and skills to care for the veteran population.

CONFLICT OF INTEREST

There are no known financial, affiliation, relationships, and activity conflicts of interest for all listed authors.

FUNDING

This work was supported by a Research and Evaluation in Residence grant (#CIN14-257) awarded by the Office of Research and Development Service and the OAA, US Department of Veterans Affairs. The views expressed here are those of the authors and do not necessarily reflect the position or policy of the US Department of Veterans Affairs or the US government.

DATA SHARING

The listed authors had full access to all of the data in the study and take responsibility for the integrity of the data and the accuracy of the data analyses.

REFERENCES

1. American Hospital Association. 2022 Health care talent scan. Chicago (IL): American Hospital Association; 2021.
2. American Association of Critical-Care Nurses. AACN guiding principles for appropriate staffing. 2018. Available at: https://www.aacn.org/policy-and-advocacy/guiding-principles-for-staffing. Accessed January 25, 2022.
3. Casey K, Oja KJ, Makic MBF. The lived experiences of graduate nurses transitioning to professional practice during a pandemic. Nurs Outlook 2021;69:1072–80.
4. Sandler M. Why are new graduate nurses leaving the profession in their first year of practice and how does this impact on ED nurse staffing? A rapid review of current literature and recommended reading. Can J Emerg Nurs 2018;41:23–4.
5. Kluwer W. Recruiting & retaining new nurse grads 2022. Available at: https://www.wolterskluwer.com/en/expert-insights/recruiting-retaining-new-nurse-grads. Accessed January 25, 2022.
6. Nursing Solutions Inc. 2021 NSI national health care retention & RN staffing report. East Petersburg, Pennsylvania: Nursing Solutions Inc.; 2021.
7. Kelly LA, Gee PM, Butler RJ. Impact of nurse burnout on organizational and position turnover. Nurs Outlook 2021;69:96–102.
8. Institute of Medicine (US). Committee on the robert wood johnson foundation initiative on the future of nursing, at the Institute of medicine. The future of nursing: leading change, advancing health. Washington (DC): National Academies Press; 2011.
9. Stephenson JK, Cosme S. Instruments to evaluate nurse residency programs: a review of the literature. J Nurses Prof Dev 2018;34:123–32.
10. Boyer SA, Valdez-Delgado KK, Huss JL, et al. Impact of a nurse residency program on transition to specialty practice. J Nurses Prof Dev 2017;33:220–7.
11. Department of Veterans Affairs. Veterans health issues related to service history. Washington (DC): Department of Veterans Affairs. Available at: https://www.va.gov/health-care/health-needs-conditions/health-issues-related-to-service-era/
12. Olenick M, Flowers M, Diaz VJ. US veterans and their unique issues: enhancing health care professional awareness. Adv Med Educ Pract 2015;6:635–9.
13. Department of Veterans Affairs. VA utilization profile FY2017. Office of data governance and analytics. National Center for Veterans Analysis and Statistics; 2020.
14. Public Law 115-182 115th congress. VA mission act of 2018. PUBL182.PS (congress.gov). Available at: https://www.congress.gov/115/plaws/publ182/PLAW-115publ182.pdf. Accessed on November 20, 2021.
15. Benner P. From novice to expert: excellence and power in clinical nursing practice. Hoboken (NJ): Prentice Hall; 1984.
16. Wagner LM, Dolansky MA, Englander R. Entrustable professional activities for quality and patient safety. Nurs Outlook 2018;66:237–43.
17. Rekman J, Gofton W, Dudek N, et al. Entrustability scales: outlining their usefulness for competency-based clinical assessment. Acad Med 2016;91:186–90.
18. Casey K, Fink R, Krugman M, et al. The graduate nurse experience. J Nurs Adm 2004;34:303–11.
19. Krippendorff K. Content analysis. In: Barnouw E, Gerbner G, Schramm W, et al, editors. International encyclopedia of communication. Oxford (UK): Oxford University Press; 1989. p. 403–7.
20. National Academy of Medicine. The future of nursing 2020-2030: charting a path to achieve health equity. Washington, DC: The National Academies; 2021.

21. American Association of Colleges of Nursing. The essentials: core competencies for professional nursing education. Washington (DC): American Association of Colleges of Nursing; 2021.
22. American Nurses Association. Nursing: scope and standards of practice. Maryland (USA): American Nurses Association; 2021.
23. American Nurses Association. Code of ethics for nurses with interpretive statements. Maryland, US: American Nurses Association; 2015.
24. Burkhart L, Bretschneider A, Gerc S, et al. Spiritual care in nursing practice in veteran health care. Glob Qual Nurs Res 2019;6.
25. Barnett P, Barnett M, Borgueta E, et al. COVID-19: an organizational-theory-guided holistic self-caring and resilience project. J Holist Nurs 2021;39:325–35.
26. Watson J. Nursing: the philosophy and science of caring. Colorado (USA): University Press of Colorado; 2008.
27. Desmond MB, Burkhart L, Horsley TL, et al. Development and psychometric evaluation of a spiritual care simulation and companion performance checklist for a veteran using a standardized patient. Clin Simul Nurs 2018;14:29–44.

Promoting Health Equity in the Latinx Community, Locally and Globally

The Duke University School of Nursing Model

Rosa M. Gonzalez-Guarda, PhD, MPH, RN, CPH, FAAN[a,b,*], Irene C. Felsman, DNP, MPH, RN[a,c], Rosa M. Solorzano, MPH, MD[a,d]

KEYWORDS

- Hispanic/Latino • Health equity • Community engagement • Nursing education
- Nursing research

KEY POINTS

- The Latinx population in the United States is the largest racial and ethnic minoritized group in the United States that experiences significant health disparities.
- Schools of nursing can play an important role in promoting health equity among Latinx communities through their academic missions of education, research, and service.
- Principles of community engagement can be implemented and combined with the cultural values important to partnering Latinx communities to foster trustworthiness.
- Programs and activities that provide learners with opportunities to partner with community and faith-based organizations to address prioritized health needs and develop skills in Spanish and cultural humility, community engaged research that informs interventions to promote health equity, and partnerships with multiple stakeholders can be led by schools of nurses to promote health equity and population health.

INTRODUCTION

The Latinx (gender inclusive term for individuals of Hispanic or Latin American descent)[1] population is a heterogenous community representing a large segment of the US population.[2] This ethnic minoritized group represents diverse racial identities, languages (including indigenous languages), heritages, immigration status, accultura-tion levels, and other social determinants that influence their health. As a whole, the

[a] Duke University School of Nursing, 307 Trent Drive, Durham, NC 27710, USA; [b] Duke Clinical Translational Science Institute, 200 Morris Street, 3rd Floor, Durham, NC 27701, USA; [c] Duke Global Health Institute, 310 Trent Drive, Durham, NC 27710, USA; [d] Duke University Romance Studies SLP, 413 Chapel Drive, Durham, NC 27708, USA
* Corresponding author. 307 Trent Drive, Durham, NC 27710.
E-mail address: rosa.gonzalez-guarda@duke.edu

Nurs Clin N Am 57 (2022) 393–411
https://doi.org/10.1016/j.cnur.2022.04.006
nursing.theclinics.com

Abbreviations	
HIV	Human Immunodificiency Virus
COVID-19	SARS-CoV2
LATIN-19	Latinx Advocacy Team and Interdisciplinary Network for COVID-19
SER	Salud/Health, Estres/Stress, y/and Resiliencia/Resilience
ICU	Intensive Care Unit
CPR	Cardiopulmonary resuscitation
ADA	American Diabetes Association

Latinx community represents 18.7% of the total US population,[3,4] with Mexican (61.5%), Puerto Rican (9.7%), Cuban (3.9%), Salvadoran (3.9%), and Dominican Republic (3.4%), representing the largest subgroups based on origin. Latinxs are among the fastest growing minoritized groups in the United States and are expected to represent 60% of the population by 2060.[5] In order to advance population health in the United States, it is imperative that nurses address the unique needs and strengths of this population. Schools of nursing across the country can play a unique role in leading efforts to promote health and well-being in this population through preparing a culturally humble nursing workforce, research that informs interventions and policies promoting health equity for this population, and providing direct services that are responsive to the needs, preferences, and strengths of the community. The purpose of this article is to describe a model used by a school of nursing for engaging and promoting health equity among the Latinx community in North Carolina.

HEALTH DISPARITIES IN THE LATINX COMMUNITY

The Latinx community in the United States experiences significant health disparities related to a myriad of health conditions. For example, when comparted with Non-Latinx White individuals, Latinx people are 23% more likely to be obese,[6] 2.5 more likely to have undiagnosed diabetes,[7] 35% more likely to have chronic liver disease,[8] and 3.6 times more likely to acquire human immunodificiency virus (HIV).[9] These health disparities are exacerbated by the fact that this group has the highest uninsurance rates in the United States,[10] significantly limiting access to needed preventative services and lifesaving treatments. For example, although Latinx individuals are less likely to have heart disease, they are more likely to have uncontrolled hypertension.[6] Latinx individuals also have lower cancer screening behaviors, placing them at risk for detecting cancer at later stages in progression.[6,11,12] Lack of insurance, interacts with other social factors such as low education levels, high rates of poverty, exposure to poor working conditions, and experiences with discrimination to place this community at a disproportionate risk for poor health.[6,13] Disparities experienced by the Latinx community became very apparent during the COVID-19 pandemic because they were 3 times more likely to acquire the infection and 2 times more likely to die than their non-Latinx White counterparts. In fact, the Latinx community has experienced a higher decline in life expectancy than non-Latinx Black and non-Latinx White individuals (3.88, 3.25, and 1.36 years, respectively) during the past 2 years.[14] If disparities among the Latinx community are not addressed, these will only continue to grow alongside the growth in this population.

Health care in the United States is not typically designed to meet the needs of the Latinx community. Not only are services often out of reach for Latinx families due to lack of insurance or proximity of these service[15,16] but they are often not culturally and linguistically tailored for this population. For example, only 7.4% of registered nurses and 6.5% of physicians are Latinx, and only a small segment of health-care providers speak Spanish, the most common language spoken by individual with Limited English Proficiency (LEP).[17–20] Although access to interpreters are required through the Culturally and Linguistically Appropriate Services (CLAS) standards, Latinx patients with LEP often have to rely on family, friends, or other untrained individuals as interpreters.[20,21] Additionally, core cultural norms and experiences are often not considered. For example, although acculturative stress, the stress associated with being Latinx in the United States and adapting to a new context, and the acculturation gaps between parents and children are key social determinants of health for Latinx families, they are rarely considered in a clinical encounter or in population health approaches targeting this population.[22–24]

The Latinx community in the US South is particularly marginalized due to systemic causes. Because the US South is a more recent immigrant-receiving region, there are less resources available for immigrants, the vast majority who are Latinx.[25] Additionally, states in the US South are among those with the highest uninsurance rates, which is in part due to the states not expanding Medicaid expansion.[16,26] Additionally, hostility toward immigrant and Latinx populations, and the adoption of community-based immigration and custom enforcement programs has contributed to fear in this populations and reluctance of Latinx immigrants to access needed health and social services.[27–31] Given this context, it is imperative that nurses go beyond the walls of their institutions to address the evolving needs of the Latinx community, leveraging strengths that exist in the culture and local context. Partnerships with trusted community-based organizations (CBOs) and faith-based organizations (FBOs) are essential in meeting the needs of this population. Duke University School of Nursing (DUSON) provides a model that is responsive to the recommendation from *The Future of Nursing 2020-2030 Charting a Path to Achieve Health Equity*[17] report and provides an exemplar of nurses leading health equity for the Latinx community.

THE DUKE UNIVERSITY SCHOOL OF NURSING LATINX ENGAGEMENT AND EQUITY MODEL

Principles

The DUSON Latinx Engagement and Equity model is built on the principles of community engagement, including principles of community engaged research (CEnR) that have been demonstrated to have an impact on promoting health equity in historically marginalized populations.[32,33]

Collaborative partnerships with diverse community organizations and leaders to address historically marginalized Latinx groups across the life span. DUSON has developed partnership with several community organizations (**Table 1**) that spans over 25 years to mirror Latinx population growth in Durham, NC, where Duke University is located (**Fig. 1**). These partnerships were developed with the intention of reaching the most historically marginalized groups in the Latinx community, such as families with a low income, uninsured individuals, and undocumented individuals who often do not seek health care within the walls of Duke Health. These organizations include both CBO and FBO, as well as community-based health-care institutions such as federally qualified health centers that provide direct clinical care. DUSON works in partnership with these organizations, never on their own, to reach a diverse population of Latinx communities across the life span and through diverse health delivery models.

Ongoing engagement that is responsive to evolving needs and opportunities. DUSON has had a long history of engaging with the Latinx community that began in 1997 in collaboration with El Centro Hispano, the first Latinx serving CBO in the region as depicted in see **Fig. 1**. This ongoing engagement has been responsive to the

Table 1
Summary of Community Organizations Duke University School of Nursing has partnered with to engaged the Latinx population

Organization	Population	Service Provided	Description of Partnership Activities
Church World Services	Immigrants and refugees	Relocation support; job preparation	• DUSON student volunteers provide safety inspection on new housing, first aid kits, and assisting families to access health care
Curamericas	Mothers and children in Latin America; Latinx in NC	Global and public health services	• Partnered on a CEnR application to test a multilevel intervention addressing acculturative stress and resilience in the Latinx immigrant population • ABSN student placements contribute to global missions and local COVID-19 response
Durham Public Schools	Latinx children	Learning together program	• ABSN clinical placements provide health education and health fairs
El Centro Hispano	Uninsured Latinx population	Health and social services, advocacy, education, English literacy	• Partner on CEnR studies to examine the effects of acculturative stress and resilience on Latinx immigrant health and to develop and test CHW delivered interventions • ABSN clinical placements contribute to their health programming
EL Futuro	Uninsured Latinx populations	Mental health services	• Placed Psychiatric Mental Health Nursing Students for clinical placements • Partnered on a CEnR application to improve the participation of Latinx in clinical trials

			• Faculty and staff volunteered at events and served on the board of directors
Iglesia la Semilla	Methodist Latinx community	Religious services; health ministry	• DUSON collaborates in COVID-19 response to provide education, testing, and vaccination • Partnered on a CEnR application to improve the participation of Latinx in clinical trials • Collaborating to develop training for CHWs and medical Spanish for students
Immaculate Conception Church	Catholic Latinx community	Religious services; health ministry; community outreach	• ABSN clinical placements and provide health education and screening after masses and facilitate support groups; CPR and first aid training for ushers.
Lincoln Community Health Center	Uninsured Latinx population	Primary health care	• D-CHIPP scholars address prioritized areas for quality improvement • Diabetes support groups in Spanish Certified Diabetes Health Educator (ADA certified) • Direct clinical care by DUSON faculty
Mexican Consulate	Mexican immigrants	Consulate services to citizens of Mexico	• ABSN students placements contribute to "la *ventanilla de salud*/the health window" providing health education and screening

Note: CEnR, community engaged research; CHW, community health workers; DUSON, Duke University School of Nursing; D-CHIPP, Community Health Improvement Partnership Program; ABSN, Accelerated Bachelor of Science in Nursing.

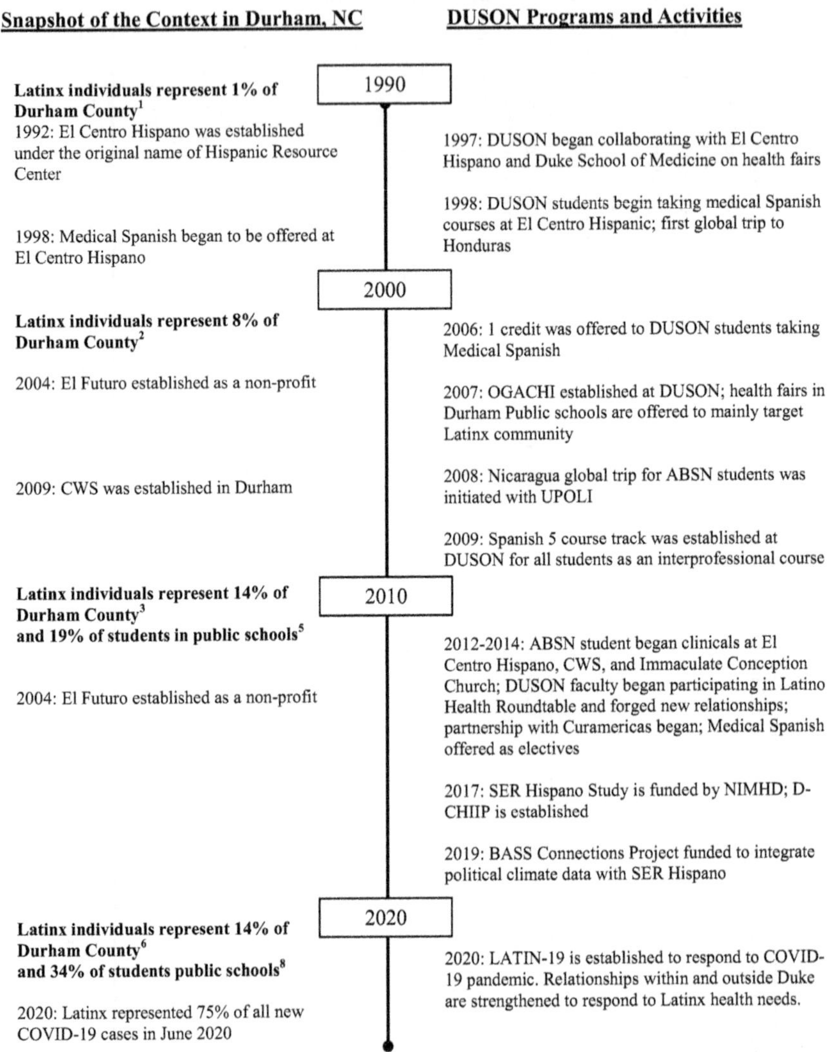

Snapshot of the Context in Durham, NC
DUSON Programs and Activities
1990
Latinx individuals represent 1% of Durham County[1]
1992: El Centro Hispano was established under the original name of Hispanic Resource Center
1997: DUSON began collaborating with El Centro Hispano and Duke School of Medicine on health fairs
1998: DUSON students begin taking medical Spanish courses at El Centro Hispanic; first global trip to Honduras
1998: Medical Spanish began to be offered at El Centro Hispano
2000
Latinx individuals represent 8% of Durham County[2]
2006: 1 credit was offered to DUSON students taking Medical Spanish
2004: El Futuro established as a non-profit
2007: OGACHI established at DUSON; health fairs in Durham Public schools are offered to mainly target Latinx community
2009: CWS was established in Durham
2008: Nicaragua global trip for ABSN students was initiated with UPOLI
2009: Spanish 5 course track was established at DUSON for all students as an interprofessional course
2010
Latinx individuals represent 14% of Durham County[3] and 19% of students in public schools[5]
2012-2014: ABSN student began clinicals at El Centro Hispano, CWS, and Immaculate Conception Church; DUSON faculty began participating in Latino Health Roundtable and forged new relationships; partnership with Curamericas began; Medical Spanish offered as electives
2004: El Futuro established as a non-profit
2017: SER Hispano Study is funded by NIMHD; D-CHIIP is established
2019: BASS Connections Project funded to integrate political climate data with SER Hispano
2020
Latinx individuals represent 14% of Durham County[6] and 34% of students public schools[8]
2020: LATIN-19 is established to respond to COVID-19 pandemic. Relationships within and outside Duke are strengthened to respond to Latinx health needs.
2020: Latinx represented 75% of all new COVID-19 cases in June 2020

Fig. 1. History of DUSON's Engagement with the Latinx community.

evolving needs of the population by making sure to (1) prioritize addressing health conditions that disproportionately impact the Latinx community, (2) being responsive to priorities identified by community organizations and coalitions, and (3) leveraging the community leaders, organizations, and networks that already exist to address these issues. For example, DUSON faculty, staff, and students engage in several health education and community-screening activities in collaboration with CBO and FBO partners to address the high levels of obesity and diabetes in the community, conditions that are not only documented to disproportionately impact the Latinx community[15] but also identified as a local community priority.[34] When the COVID-19 pandemic affected the globe and was at its peak, affecting 3 times as many Latinx individuals than non-Latinx whites,[35] DUSON responded to this disparity by deploying bilingual/bicultural nursing students as part of the contact tracers in partnerships with organization who were leading this such a Curamerica, conducting research to understand drivers of this disparities and potential solutions through an existing study funded through the National Institutes of Health (R01MD012249), and partnered with a coalition of multiple stakeholder to advocate for Latinx health equity during the pandemic. The ongoing engagement of DUSON with the Latinx community, pre-pandemic, facilitated the success of advocacy efforts.

Spanning the tripartite mission of education, research, and service to enhance mutual benefits. The DUSON model intentionally spans the academic missions of education, research, and service. This has helped ensure that there is mutual benefit from both the community and academic stakeholder and created a balance between research and action. For example, faculty and staff meet monthly with leaders from El Centro Hispano's health program. In those meetings, faculty and staff check in on the progress related to a collaborative CEnR study, plan community, and public health clinical activities that are responsive to the organization's and community needs and assess organizational needs from both the community and academic perspective. The clinical placements of student at El Centro allows DUSON to offer assistance to El Centro in meeting their goals for their health program through the support of the students, providing a benefit for El Centro and a service for the community while simultaneously providing training experiences for students. The provision of health services such as evidence-based education and screening while data are still being collected and analyzed from a separate research study allows DUSON to provide care while new interventions are being developed and tested through research. Partner needs are also addressed and have resulted in mutual benefits. For example, El Centro has asked DUSON faculty and staff to provide training to their staff (eg, mental health education for community health workers [CHWs]) and DUSON faculty and staff have asked El Centro to conduct trainings on the local Latinx community for learners.

Diverse representation from both Latinx and non-Latinx nurses and interdisciplinary partners that fosters cultural humility. The DUSON model intentionally engages faculty, students, and staff from diverse heritages, immigration and generational experiences, racial and gender identities, and language preferences in addressing the needs to the Latinx community. The model intentionally engages both bilingual and bicultural health care providers and individuals from non-Latinx identities in this study, recognizing the importance for all health-care providers to have a level of awareness of the needs and strengths of the Latinx community. The diverse learning and working environment helps to foster the actions that come from the Rainbow Model of Cultural Humility (eg, openness, self-awareness, flexibility, recognition of power imbalance),[36] to support each other to tailor responses to the population, avoid stereotypes and biases, and serve as advocates for change in health-care institutions. For example, in the Medical Spanish courses that are provided, learners from diverse personal identities and disciplines to engage in bidirectional learning in partnership with community partners who contribute to an understanding of how the local context shapes the experience of diverse local Latinx communities and helps inform tailored approaches that are responsive.

Respeto and Carino as Core values. Respeto (respect) and *Cariño* (love) are core values for many Latinx communities that are vital for health promoting interactions with health-care providers.[37,38] The DUSON Model intentionally incorporates these values in our approach through specific behaviors demonstrated to the community. Respect is operationalized in a multitude ways. DUSON faculty, staff, and students do not engage with the Latinx community without a CBO or FBO partner that has established trustworthiness in the community. Value is also placed on the lived experience of the community and their expertise. For example, DUSON faculty, staff, and students often work with CHWs to design, implement, and evaluate health initiatives. Every individual is treated with the dignity they deserve and services are provided despite access to documents that are often required in health care such as a license and a health insurance card. For example, in a CEnR research study led by DUSON addressing the Latinx community, investigators were able to get a waiver for collecting social security numbers or tax identification to compensate participants for their participation. *Cariño* is approached through communicating warmth as interpersonal relationships are established and care is provided. This can be demonstrated by gestures that can range from asking for aspects of the individual's personal life such as their family demonstrating a connection such as a common heritage, providing a card with a personal message (eg, birthday cards for research participants), and expressing affection during interactions such as engaging in an embrace when a patient expressed gratitude for providing health service. These culturally responsive strategies are foundational to establishing trustworthiness with this population.[39]

Institutional support for Latinx Engagement. Institutional support by DUSON and the broader Duke University community has helped facilitate meaningful and sustainable engagement with the Latinx community. DUSON's Office of Global and Community Health Affairs facilitated early engagement with the Latinx community, both locally and globally. In 2017, the DUSON Community Health Improvement Partnership Program (D-CHIPP) was established and provided additional infrastructure and funding to support local community engagement as a result of the implementation of the school strategic plan. For example, through funding provided by D-CHIPP, DUSON was able to purchase hemoglobin A1C screening materials to expand diabetes screening in the Latinx community and in accordance to established guidelines.[40] DUSON's Center for Nursing Research has helped provide training for community partners in submitting grants and supported an institutional license to be able to make the collaborative institutional training initiative (CITI)[41] available in Spanish. The Community Engaged Research Initiative (CERI) of the Duke Clinical Translational Institute provides additional support through consultations, education/training, providing funding, supporting community coalitions, and advocacy to support CEnR. For example, CERI has helped facilitate community consultation studios for DUSON faculty. These consultation studios are on the engagement studio model[42] and have provided opportunities for DUSON faculty engaged in research with the Latinx community to receive their input on their research ideas and protocols. DUSON has also worked with Duke's Office of Civic Engagement to broker relationships between Duke University and Latinx serving organizations to respond to emerging needs such as the mental health crises that has been exacerbated in the Latinx community by the pandemic. This tapestry of services provides a rich environment for engagement.

Core Programs and Activities

DUSON has core programs with a specific focus on engagement with the Latinx community that builds on its academic, research, and service missions. These programs are integrated in the 5 academic programs: Accelerated Bachelor of Science in Nursing (ABSN); Master of Science in Nursing (MSN), which include 8 advanced practice nursing specialties and 3 nonclinical majors; Doctor of Nursing Practice (DNP), inclusive of a Certified Registered Nurse Anesthetists (CRNA) tract, and a PhD program. Three of these are onsite (ABSN, CRNA, PhD), allowing for the opportunity for students to be immersed in work in the local Latinx community.

ABSN Local Community Clinical Immersion Experiences. The ABSN program includes a community and public health required course with 56 hours of clinical immersion. Groups of 6–10 students are imbedded in various CBOs and FBOs with long-standing engagement with DUSON (see **Table 1**). Students with Spanish language ability (beginner, proficient, or native speakers) work with bilingual/bicultural instructors to (1) conduct a community assessment (windshield/walking surveys; key informant interviews; focus groups surveys), identifying assets and needs; (2) determine mutual goals and objectives with community partners; (3) plan an intervention; (4) and finally evaluating the success of the programming. Examples of areas of intervention include hypertension, diabetes, obesity, nutrition and food insecurity, infectious disease (HIV and COVID-19), hygiene, women's health, and stress and resilience, all health disparities prioritized by the Latinx local community.

ABSN Global Clinical Immersion Experiences. A percentage of ABSN students opt to fulfill their community and public health clinical hours through a global immersion program offered as an alternative to the local experience. Groups of up to 10 students travel with an experienced clinical instructor to one of several Latin American countries, including Nicaragua, Guatemala, and Honduras, regions that represent the origins of a significant proportion of the local Latinx community in Durham, NC. Students in the Global Immersion carrying out similar activities as the local immersion, however, within the context of a different health system and culture that helps facilitate their understanding of the lived experiences of immigrants in the United States as they encounter a new context.

Masters, PhD, and DNP Student Clinical Placements and Engagement. Graduate level students often leverage the faculty's long-standing community partnerships with the Latinx community for research and quality improvement projects. For example, one longitudinal study of Latinx young adults has allowed students in several programs to learn about CEnR and contribute to data collection, analyses, and dissemination. These have been used as Directed Scholarship opportunities (independent studies), research practicum, and dissertation research. In addition, through a university wide funding source [Bass connections], students from the undergraduate to PhD levels have had the opportunity to work with faculty and postdoctoral fellows on several focused research projects pertaining to the Latinx community. When MSN students are local, they can be placed in local settings serving the Latinx community such as clinical placement at El Futuro for students in the Psychiatric Mental Health Nursing postmasters certificate program. Several DNP quality improvement scholarly projects have focused on the Latinx population, in South America and in North Carolina. Two projects in Bolivia addressed triage protocols in an outpatient clinic and another on appropriate diagnosis of bacterial infection and antibiotic prescription.[43] An NC project focused on diabetes peer education within the Latinx community.

Volunteer Opportunities. Outside of the formal academic program, nursing students at all levels have several volunteer service opportunities that they may choose to be involved in. In the local community, an annual Latinx health fair is organized by El Centro Hispano with support from DUSON and other community partners. Nursing students and other learners (eg, Medical Spanish) participate in screenings, health education, and triage activities. Throughout the pandemic, students have volunteered in COVID testing and vaccination efforts through various community-organized events. A student club, Nursing Students Without Borders, engages in service to the Latinx community, both locally and globally. They partner with a local resettlement organization (Church World Service) to prepare housing for new immigrant families, including doing a safety inspection, providing first aid kits, and assisting families to access health care. Students collaborate with a faculty advisor to organize an annual service trip to the Guatemalan highlands to work with midwives and health workers in a remote community-based health center focused on maternal-child survival. Nursing alumni, as well as other health professional students often join students on this trip.

Interprofessional Courses in Medical Spanish. Medical Spanish and Cultural Competence courses started at DUSON in 1998 as an interprofessional initiative funded by the Duke Endowment that also engaged different departments at Duke (Physician Assistant, Physical Therapy, and Medical Students, Residency Programs), the Linguistic Center at El Centro Hispano, and Lincoln Community Center. These courses have evolved from evening classes offered at El Centro Hispano for no credit, to a series of courses that are offered for credit that includes distance-based components delivered through synchronous and asynchronous activities. Currently, Medical Spanish courses are offered through 2 3-credit hour elective courses tailored for both beginners and advanced learners (see curriculum on **Table 2**). Nursing students from different levels of experience and across academic programs at DUSON bring their unique perspectives to embrace cultural diversity, respect the unique perspectives of other disciplines within their own body of practice, whereas contributing to the needs of the team. Such a meaningful collaboration allows students to engage others through joint didactic classwork, which permits them to delineate individuals' roles and responsibilities serving as a model for future patient care to maintain their own competence in their profession.[40]

A myriad of teaching and learning strategies are integrated with synchronous and asynchronous strategies to enhance competency in Medial Spanish and interprofessional care for Spanish-speaking communities. Simulation activities (eg, providing labor and delivery and postpartum care to a family) are integrated into the course, and students are allowed to apply their medical Spanish speaking skills to gain confidence and receive appropriate feedback when errors ensue within the context of their role on the interprofessional team. Distance-based students are able to participate through video conference throughout the simulation. These courses also offer students local and global opportunities where students can practice in "real world" settings through community experiences such as participating in a health fair in collaboration with El Centro Hispano or participating in a global immersion trip. Finally, students are paired with students from la *Universidad Politécnica de Nicaragua*/the Polytechnical University of Nicaragua University, Nicaragua and engage in 3 conversations, were they share experiences about their culture, nursing profession while practicing their Spanish oral skills. DUSON students also have the opportunity to participate every year in the interprofessional course and clinical outreach Exploring Medicine: Cross-Cultural Challenges to Health in the 21 Century-Honduras. The team consists of faculty, staff, and students from the Schools of Nursing and Medicine. During the course and outreach, students learn about how culture influences the delivery of health care, provide health education, and basic clinical and dental care to a rural Honduran community. The team works very closely with the Honduran health system and CBO whom identify their needs. Lessons learned from the trip are translated to their care of Latinx families in the local communities.

Research addressing Latinx Health Equity. In 2017, the SER (*Salud, Estrés, y Resiliencia*/Stress, Health and Resilience) Hispano study was funded by the National Institute on Minority Health and Health Disparities (R01MD012249, PI: Gonzalez-Guarda, R.M.) to examine the Impact of acculturative stress and resilience on the syndemic outcome of substance abuse, violence, HIV, and mental health as well as stress biomarkers. This was the first research study at DUSON specifically addressing health equity in the local Latinx community. This initial funding was leveraged to enhance the scope of this research to include examining the impact of the political climate on the health (Bass Connections Grant; PIs: Stafford, A., Nagy, G., & Felsman, I.), to engage the community in identifying needs and preferences for interventions

Table 2
Medical Spanish and cultural competence curriculum

	Introduction to Medical Spanish and Cultural Competence Level I and II	Advanced Medical Spanish and Cultural Competence Levels I and II
Course Description	Designed to help health-care professionals and learners develop basic languages skills in Medical Spanish to enhance their cultural competence when caring for Latinx patients. Aspects of Latin American culture—especially those most pertinent to health care—are included in each lesson	Designed to help students achieve fluency when engaged in health-related interactions with Latin American populations. Aspects of Latin American culture—especially those most pertinent to health care—are addresses as students engage in more complex or emotionally charged interactions with the Latinx population
Delivery	12 sessions 1:45 min synchronous/ 1:45 min asynchronous work	12 sessions 1:45 min synchronous/ 1:45 min asynchronous work
Objectives	1. Use basic sentences in present tense, past and future tenses of regular and irregular verbs for common health-related patient care issues 2. Use medical Spanish vocabulary in patient-related situations, such as intake or health history interviews, conducting a physical examination or providing health-related education to Latinx populations 3. Explain unique considerations health providers must make to respect cultural beliefs and practices when conducting intake or health history interviews with Latin American patients/families 4. Explain unique considerations health providers must make to respect cultural beliefs and practices	1. Communicate in Spanish using fluent language skills (written, oral, reading, listening) incorporating the present tense, present perfect, past, imperfect mood of the past and future tenses of regular verbs and other common health related reflexive and irregular verbs 2. Engage in dialog with Latinx patients/families about health-related issues or decisions using fluent Spanish language skills and medical vocabulary 3. Explain unique considerations health providers must make to respect cultural beliefs and practices when engaging in dialogue about health-related issues or decisions with Latin American patients/families 4. Use medical Spanish vocabulary in the context of simulated patient care scenarios on nursing care skills 5. Correctly convey Spanish speaking Latin American patient's questions and concerns about health care to non-Spanish speaking health providers

(*continued on next page*)

Table 2
(*continued*)

	Introduction to Medical Spanish and Cultural Competence Level I and II	Advanced Medical Spanish and Cultural Competence Levels I and II
		6. Explain unique considerations health providers must make to respect cultural beliefs and practices when performing nursing care skills and using an interpreter with Latin American patients/families
Content	Level I • *Verbs:* To be (Ser and Estar), to have (tener), to hurt/pain (dolor/doler) • *Grammar:* Verbs in present tense, regular verbs and some irregular verbs, past participate as an adjective, basic sentence structure, making questions • *Vocabulary:* Medical professions and specialties, countries of origin, symptoms, injuries, body parts and organs, days of the week, numbers, clinic items, vital signs, family, pharmacy, taking a basic interview-intake form • *Cultural Competence:* basics, family, attitudes toward health care, impact on effective communication with health-care providers, social drivers of health Level II • *Verbs:* Verbs gustar, querer, preferir, deber, regular verbs for the physical examination • *Grammar*: present tense, future tense, past tense, direct and indirect object pronoun • *Vocabulary:* Diet and Nutrition, health history, physical examination, illnesses and symptoms, cardiovascular, maternity, mental health, infectious diseases • *Cultural Competence*: Cultural thoughts and attitudes toward traditional medicine, nutrition, mental health, and childbearing. Practicing interview models applying	Level I • *Verbs*: To be (Ser and Estar), to have (tener), Pain (dolor/doler) • *Grammar*: Verbs in present tense, regular and some irregular verbs, past participate, future sentence, basic sentence structure, elaborating questions • *Vocabulary*: Medical Professions and specialties, Countries of origin, symptoms, injuries, body parts and organs, days of the week, clinic items, vital signs, family, pharmacy, conducting a medical interview-intake form, introduction to the physical examination, some illnesses • *Oral Skills*: Conduct a medical interview using numbers, day of the week, key question, and commands for physical examination. Provide education about and medications in Spanish • *Cultural Competence*: basics principles of cultural competence, family, pharmacy/traditional medicine and attitudes toward health care Level II • *Verbs*: reflexive verbs, regular, and irregular verbs, commands • *Grammar*: past and present perfect tense, imperfect mood of the past tense, future tense • *Vocabulary*: Nutrition, Physical examination, test and procedures, hospital admissions and presurgery care, illnesses and review of systems, how to become an interpreter, basics skills in nursing

(*continued on next page*)

Table 2
(*continued*)

	Introduction to Medical Spanish and Cultural Competence Level I and II	Advanced Medical Spanish and Cultural Competence Levels I and II
	concepts of humility, respect, and personalism relevant to the Latino culture. Roles of the interpreter/patient/provider	• *Oral Skills*: Conduct a complete health interview using symptoms, diseases, systems, medical procedures. Provide education about nutrition, medications, maternity, trauma, mental health. Conduct basic nursing skills with focus on giving education in Spanish using the simulation laboratory • *Cultural Competence*: Cultural thoughts and attitudes toward traditional medicine, nutrition, mental health, and childbearing. Practicing interview models applying concepts of humility, respect, and personalism relevant to the Latino culture. Roles of the interpreter/patient/provider
Evaluation methods	• Homework • Quizzes/Examinations • Oral video recordings • Class Participation	• Homework • Quizzes/Examinations • Oral video recordings • Class Participation • Essays

addressing acculturative stress (diversity supplement, Nagy, G.), and pilot different approaches using a multitude of funding available through Duke. CEnR strategies were integrated throughout these studies and included community partners as coinvestigators and members of the research team, consultants of the research (eg, community consultation studios, advisory boards), the use of bicultural and bilingual members of the local community such as CHWs as interventionists, and a focus on returning the results to the participants through newsletters and events that allowed participants and health and social providers to come together, entitled "Access to Immigrants." Research from this team has helped advocate for the Latinx community during the COVID-19 pandemic, and served as a source of training for learners from a range of disciplines (eg, nursing, medicine, psychology, global health, anthropology) and levels of training (eg, undergraduate to postdoctoral). A Latinx health equity laboratory has also been established at DUSON to support a growing community of scholars that are addressing diverse health equity topics in their research in partnership with Latinx communities.

The Latinx Advocacy and Interdisciplinary Network for COVID-19 (LATIN-19). DUSON faculty, staff, and students have been key leaders of LATIN-19, is a coalition of more than 700 registrants that have convened since the onset of the COVID-19 pandemic to focus on strategies for reducing health disparities in the Latinx community during COVID-19.[44] Members of LATIN-19 represent diverse sectors including health care, public health, CBOs, FBOs, education, government, media, and others. Members of the DUSON community collaborate with this extensive network through their service on the executive team, helping to lead events such as vaccination clinics, supporting staffing events with trained bilingual/bicultural student volunteers (eg, ABSN students with local and global placements serving the Latinx community; Medical Spanish students), and leading research and evaluation efforts for the coalition.

The coalition leverages the strength of preexisting community partnerships and fosters new collaborations among community members with a commitment to the Latinx population.[13] About 60 to 100 participants meet weekly via a virtual platform. The weekly meeting allows for information sharing from diverse perspective, opportunities to network and collaborate, and the opportunity for individuals in leadership positions to listen directly from community members on their lived experiences during the pandemic. Hearing stories directly from community members has been a key driver to promote change and action around issues regarding the health of the Latinx community. Simultaneous interpretation is provided in English and Spanish. The LATIN-19 approach uses the principles of the socio-ecological model (eg, intrapersonal, interpersonal, community levels, and so forth) of health and community engagement to respond to the unique needs of the Latinx community.[45] Interventions by Latin-19 include creation and dissemination of health promotion materials through partner organizations, coordination of testing and vaccine clinics, production of public service announcements, engagement with media across multiple platforms to create awareness of health disparities affecting the community, and advocacy for systems changes to promote health equity in this community.

IMPACT

DUSON's Model for Latinx Engagement and Health Equity is far reaching and has an impact on a learners, faculty and staff, and the broader community.

Learners

DUSON's increasing efforts to engage students in addressing the needs of the Latinx community through an equity lens have had several benefits for learners. Not the least of these is to highlight through real-time experience the importance of cultural intelligence when working with diverse individuals and families, both in their countries of origin and in their chosen country of resettlement, the United States (Buchanan and colleagues 2021). Didactic learning, coupled with clinical immersion experience, allows for integration of concepts and skills. Students learn through immersive experience essential concepts regarding global socio-political issues pertaining to the Latinx population, both locally and globally (Clarke and colleagues, 2016). Through faculty and clinical instructor guidance, students are prompted to reflect on personal expectations and cultural perspectives regarding community members and professional colleagues they interact with during immersion experiences (Onasu, 2021) and gain skills and confidence in intercultural interactions. Interprofessional learning is another benefit, illustrated by this DUSON alumni comment,

> *"My time in Honduras was an invaluable experience that I will never forget. I learned how to work on a team of inter-professional health-care members and contribute towards a diagnosis and treatment plan."*

Faculty and Staff

The long history of Latinx engagement at DUSON has helped recruit Latinx faculty, staff, and students at DUSON, demonstrating a clear commitment to promoting health equity in this population. For example, in 2016, a Latinx faculty was attracted to DUSON because an expanded strategic focus on community and population health at DUSON and an ongoing educational and service initiatives serving the Latinx population. Shortly thereafter, she received funding through NIMHD for the SER Hispano study and hired a total of 5 new staff at DUSON during the course of the project, 4 of whom continue to work at Duke through different research and clinical activities. Working in an institution that has other members of the Latinx community has helped provide a community of colleagues with similar interest, a support structure, and helped promote a sense of belonging and well-being at the school. It also serves as an approach to help begin changing practices and structures to be more inclusive. For example, as a result of the SER Hispano research team advocating for research training in Spanish (eg, CITI), the Center of Nursing Research at DUSON bought the institutional license for the modules in Spanish, allowing the entire Duke community access to these.

Community

It is the mission of DUSON faculty to work toward mutual benefit for students and community through community engaged programs, both locally and globally. Faculty members are active on boards and health department committees that carry out important clinical and public health functions (eg, inform direct mental health clinical care; community health assessments) and advance policies and enhance organizational responsiveness to the Latinx community through advocacy. DUSON's engagement with the Latinx community has grown proportionately as the Latinx population has grown during the past 30 years. Since the onset of the COVID-19 pandemic, this relationship has strengthened dramatically due to faculty, staff, and student response to efforts to mitigate the health and socioeconomic effects on this community. This engagement has not only contributed to community health improvement that resulted from changes in health-care practices (eg, more inclusive care for Latinx and Spanish speaking patients in the ICU) but also closed important gaps in vaccine inequities that existed when these first became available but then mitigated through hyperlocal strategies led by LATIN-19.[46]

CLINICS CARE POINTS

Below is a list of key strategies clinicians can implement to promote health equity in the Latinx community:

- Go beyond the walls of health-care institutions to partner with trusted CBOs and FBOs who are serving the local Latinx community.
- Assess the social determinants of health when providing care to the Latinx community, including their experiences of acculturative stress.
- Connect Latinx individuals and families with existing services in the community that address the social determinants of health.
- Ensure that referral services are available in the preferred language of your patient (eg, Spanish or indigenous language) and that those being referred are eligible for receipt of services (eg, required driver's license; health insurance).
- Advocate for Latinx and immigrant friendly environments in your practice setting, including the availability of CLAS.

SUMMARY

In order to improve population health, it is becoming increasingly vital to address evolving health disparities experienced by the Latinx community, the largest racial and ethnic minoritized community in the United States. Schools of Nursing are uniquely positioned to promote health equity in this population through their education, research, and service missions. The DUSON Model for Latinx Community Engagement and Health Equity is a comprehensive model that is responsive to the recommendations of *The Future of Nursing Report 2020-2030*[17] and include key principles of community engagement that have a strong evidence based in promoting health equity among historically marginalized communities.[33] Through innovative local and global immersion programs, service provided through volunteer work, innovative interprofessional training in Medical Spanish, CEnR to inform interventions that promote health equity, and partnerships with diverse stakeholders and sectors that go beyond health care, DUSON is having an impact on learners, the DUSON anduniversity community, the Latinx community being served, and population health more broadly. This model could be disseminated throughout other schools of nursing to inform a responsive strategy promoting health equity.

DISCLOSURE

Funding for projects being reported in this paper included research supported by the National Institute on Minority Health and Health Disparities of the National Institutes of Health under Award Number R01MD012249 and research infrastructure supported through the National Center Advancing Translation Science under Award Number 5UL1TR002553. Additional support was provided by Duke University School of Nursing and the Duke University COVID Philanthropic fund. The content is solely the responsibility of the authors and does not necessarily represent the official views ofthe National Institutes of Health or Duke University. The authors also wish to acknowledge the important contributions of the community organizations mentioned in this paper and the faculty, staff, students and community partners involved in the initiatives described.

REFERENCES

1. Salinas C Jr. The complexity of the “x” in Latinx: How Latinx/a/o students relate to, identify with, and understand the term Latinx. J Hispanic Higher Educ 2020;19(2): 149–68.
2. US Census Bureau. Quick facts: Durham County, North Carolina; United States, Population Estimates, July 1 2021, (V2021). US Census Bureau; 2022. Available at: https://www.census.gov/quickfacts/fact/table/durhamcountynorthcarolina,US/POP010210. [Accessed 5 June 2022]. Accessed June 5, 2022.
3. U.S.C. BureauQuick Facts %U. Available at: https://www.census.gov/quickfacts/fact/table/US/PST045219. Accessed June 5, 2021.
4. Schools DCP. Facts and figures about durham public schools. n.d Available at: https://www.dpsnc.net/domain/78.
5. Bureau USC. Hispanic population to reach 111 million by 2060 %U. 2018. Available at: https://www.census.gov/library/visualizations/2018/comm/hispanic-projected-pop.html.
6. Centers for Disease Control and Prevention OoMHaHE. Hispanic health. 2015. Vital Signs: Available at: https://www.cdc.gov/vitalsigns/hispanic-health/index.html. Accessed January 5, 2022.
7. Marquez I, Calman N, Crump C. A framework for addressing diabetes-related disparities in US Latino populations. J Community Health 2019;44(2):412–22.
8. Prevention CfDCa. Liver Disease. 2016.
9. Prevention CfDCa. HIV Surveillance Report. 2019.

10. Buchmueller TC, Levinson ZM, Levy HG, et al. Effect of the affordable care Act on racial and ethnic disparities in health insurance coverage. Am J Public Health 2016;106(8):1416–21.
11. Miranda PY, Tarraf W, González HM. Breast cancer screening and ethnicity in the United States: implications for health disparities research. Breast Cancer Res Treat 2011;128(2):535–42.
12. Liss DT, Baker DW. Understanding current racial/ethnic disparities in colorectal cancer screening in the United States: the contribution of socioeconomic status and access to care. Am J Prev Med 2014;46(3):228–36.
13. Martinez-Bianchi V, Panayotti GMM, Corsino L, et al. Health and wellness for our latina community: the work of the latinx advocacy team & interdisciplinary network for COVID-19 (LATIN-19). N C Med J 2021;82(4):278–81.
14. Woolf SH, Masters RK, Aron LY. Effect of the covid-19 pandemic in 2020 on life expectancy across populations in the USA and other high income countries: simulations of provisional mortality data. BMJ 2021;373:n1343.
15. Edward J, Biddle DJ. Using geographic information systems (GIS) to examine barriers to healthcare access for Hispanic and Latino immigrants in the US south. J Racial Ethnic Health Disparities 2017;4(2):297–307.
16. Keisler-Starkey K, Bunch LN. Health Insurance Coverage in the United States: 2020. Curr Popul Rep 2021;P60:274.
17. Wakefield M, Williams DR, Le Menestrel S. The future of nursing 2020-2030: charting a path to achieve health equity. Washington, DC: National Academy of Sciences; 2021.
18. Colleges AAoM. Diversity in medicine: facts and figures 2019 2022. Available at: https://www.aamc.org/data-reports/workforce/interactive-data/figure-18-percentage-all-active-physicians-race/ethnicity-2018. Accessed January 16, 2022.
19. Artiga S, Young K, Cornachione E, et al. The role of language in health care access and utilization for insured Hispanic adults. Menlo Park, CA: Henry J. Disparities Policy. Kaiser Family Foundation,; 2015.
20. Himmelstein J, Himmelstein DU, Woolhandler S, et al. Health Care Spending And Use Among Hispanic Adults With And Without Limited English Proficiency, 1999–2018: Study examines health care spending and use among Hispanic individuals with and without limited English proficiency. Health Aff 2021;40(7):1126–34.
21. Schenker Y, Pérez-Stable EJ, Nickleach D, et al. Patterns of interpreter use for hospitalized patients with limited English proficiency. J Gen Intern Med 2011; 26(7):712–7.
22. González-Guarda RM, McCabe BE, Leblanc N, et al. The contribution of stress, cultural factors, and sexual identity on the substance abuse, violence, HIV, and depression syndemic among Hispanic men. Cultur Divers Ethnic Minor Psychol 2016;22(4):563.
23. Gonzalez-Guarda RM, Stafford AM, Nagy GA, et al. A systematic review of physical health consequences and acculturation stress among Latinx individuals in the United States. Biol Res Nurs 2021;23(3):362–74.
24. Smokowski PR, Rose R, Bacallao ML. Acculturation and Latino family processes: how cultural involvement, biculturalism, and acculturation gaps influence family dynamics. Fam Relat 2008;57(3):295–308.
25. Odem ME, Lacy EC. Latino immigrants and the transformation of the US South. Athens, London: University of Georgia Press; 2009.

26. Courtemanche C, Marton J, Ukert B, et al. Early impacts of the Affordable Care Act on health insurance coverage in Medicaid expansion and non-expansion states. J Policy Anal Manage 2017;36(1):178–210.
27. Perreira KM, Pedroza JM. Policies of exclusion: implications for the health of immigrants and their children. Annu Rev Public Health 2019;40:147–66.
28. O'Neil K, Tienda M. A tale of two counties: natives' opinions toward immigration in North Carolina. Int Migr Rev 2010;44(3):728–61.
29. Weissman DM. The federalization of racism and nativist hostility: local immigration enforcement in North Carolina. In: InMigration in an era of restriction and recession 2016. Cham: Springer:99–115.
30. Mann-Jackson L, Song EY, Tanner AE, et al. The health impact of experiences of discrimination, violence, and immigration enforcement among Latino men in a new settlement state. Am J Mens Health 2018;12(6):1937–47.
31. Rhodes SD, Mann L, Simán FM, et al. The impact of local immigration enforcement policies on the health of immigrant Hispanics/Latinos in the United States. Am J Public Health 2015;105(2):329–37.
32. Blanchard L, Furco A. Faculty engaged scholarship: setting standards and building conceptual clarity. 2021. The Academy of Community Engagement Scholarship %U Available at: https://doi.org/10.17615/0xj1-c495.
33. Cyril S, Smith BJ, Possamai-Inesedy A, et al. Exploring the role of community engagement in improving the health of disadvantaged populations: a systematic review. Glob Health Action 2015;8(1):29842.
34. Durham PfH. 2020 Durham County Community Health Assessment. 2021.
35. Case demographics. North Carolina department of health and human services; 2021. Available at: https://covid19.ncdhhs.gov/dashboard/cases. Accessed April 14, 2021.
36. Foronda C. A theory of cultural humility. J Transcult Nurs 2020;31(1):7–12.
37. Calzada EJ, Fernandez Y, Cortes DE. Incorporating the cultural value of respeto into a framework of Latino parenting. Cult Divers Ethnic Minor Psychol 2010; 16(1):77.
38. Fischer SM, Kline DM, Min S-J, et al. Effect of Apoyo con Cariño (Support With Caring) trial of a patient navigator intervention to improve palliative care outcomes for Latino adults with advanced cancer: a randomized clinical trial. JAMA Oncol 2018;4(12):1736–41.
39. Fischer SM, Kline DM, Min S-J, et al. Apoyo con Carino: strategies to promote recruiting, enrolling, and retaining Latinos in a cancer clinical trial. J Natl Compr Cancer Netw 2017;15(11):1392–9.
40. Hermann CP, Head BA, Black K, et al. Preparing nursing students for interprofessional practice: the interdisciplinary curriculum for oncology palliative care education. J Prof Nurs 2016;32(1):62–71.
41. Braunschweiger P, Hansen K. Collaborative institutional training initiative (CITI). J Clin Res Best Pract 2010;6:1–6.
42. Joosten YA, Israel TL, Williams NA, et al. Community engagement studios: a structured approach to obtaining meaningful input from stakeholders to inform research. Acad Med 2015;90(12):1646.
43. Rivasplata H, Dettmann N, LeVan ER, et al. A continued professional development nursing partnership in a remote bolivian hospital. J Contin Educ Nurs 2021;52(3):142–9.
44. Krogstad JM, Gonzalez-Barrera A, Noe-Bustamante L. US Latinos among hardest hit by pay cuts, job losses due to coronavirus. Washington, DC: Pew Research Center; 2020.

45. Martinez O, Arreola S, Wu E, et al. Syndemic factors associated with adult sexual HIV risk behaviors in a sample of Latino men who have sex with men in New York City. Drug and alcohol dependence 2016;166:258–62.
46. Andrea Thoumi M, Kaalund K, Silcox C, et al. Hyperlocal covid-19 testing and vaccination strategies to reach communities with low vaccine uptake: considerations for states and localities. 2021. Available at: https://healthpolicy.duke.edu/sites/default/files/2021-09/Hyperlocal%20COVID%20Testing%20Vaccination_1.pdf.

Rural and Indigenous Vulnerable Populations

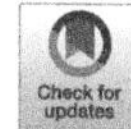

A Case Study

Lyn Behnke, DNP, FNP-BC, PMHNP-BC, CAFCI, CTEL, CHFN*

KEYWORDS

• Rural • Native American • Poverty • Health policy • Nursing education

KEY POINTS

- Intergenerational trauma can be a critical factor in developing substance use disorder.
- Many people do not realize that their substance use/abuse is generational.
- Adverse childhood events and situations contribute to poor mental health in later years.
- Health policy must be developed to facilitate the resolution of adverse social determinants of health.
- Native and rural populations develop resilience despite adverse events. The strength must be positive and taught in a culturally humble way.

INTRODUCTION/HISTORY/DEFINITIONS/BACKGROUND

Robert is a 26-year-old Native American man found unconscious in the hallway of a small apartment building in a small town in a rural northern state. Friends who were with him were hysterical over the possibility of him dying. (They used heroin as a new "shipment" that had arrived from "downstate." They had no idea that one of them may die that night.) cardiopulmonary rescusitation (CPR) was started, just compressions as no one was comfortable breathing for Robert. Fortunately, one of the participants had attended rehab "downstate" and had two doses of Narcan 4 mg.; both doses were required to bring Robert around. The group had called 911, and the State Police attended the scene and made sure that Robert was transported to the area hospital. The hospital is a critical access hospital known by the community as the "band-aid station." Robert was held in the emergency room for 72 hours as there are no inpatient substance use or psychiatric facilities in this rural tourist town. The closest psych beds are 100 miles away. The soonest psychiatric evaluation appointment was 3 months out. Robert denied being suicidal and thus was discharged from the emergency room to the county jail on drug charges.

University of Michigan – Flint, 303 East Kearsley Street, Flint, MI 48502, USA
* Corresponding author. 1115 Townline Road, Tawas City, MI 48763.
E-mail address: lynbehnke@gmail.com

Nurs Clin N Am 57 (2022) 413–420
https://doi.org/10.1016/j.cnur.2022.04.007

Robert is currently unemployed. The only employment hub involves routine drug testing, and he has been unable to pass a drug test (marijuana) for 3 years. He is currently working "under the table" at a local restaurant run by a family member, and when sober enough, he runs a saw for his grandparents.

Robert was born in 1996 and is the son of Gladys Owl, who was born in 1977, and an unknown father. Gladys was born near the native reservation in the northernmost region of the rural state. Her mother, Isa, was born on the reservation in 1959 but relocated quickly by her parents because of the initiative to remove native children from their homes and take them to schools run by religious or "humanitarian" organizations. Isa's parents were survivors of the Indian school in the northernmost region. They were forced to attend the schools until they were closed in 1970. All traditional knowledge had been expunged from their knowledge and life. They no longer practiced their native language, knew nothing of ceremonies that included healing, life transitions, birth, marriage, or death and did not know the subtle traditions of their culture as Native Americans. Isa denies that she is Native American and Gladys and Robert are Native but just poor rural people living in the north. However, their birth certificates indicate that they were born to Native parents. The tribe was not identified. Consequently, they were not eligible for tribal funding. They make their living by working in the woods, cutting, stacking, and selling timber to tourists in the summer and local families in the winter.

Gladys recently obtained a job at the new casino that opened a month ago. She is relieved to have a job, it currently pays 9.50 an hour, but now she can routinely afford food and alcohol. She lives in a cabin that she and her father built. She worked with them in the woods until the casino opened. She has been arrested for driving under the influence and being drunk and disorderly by the local officials. The tribal nations have never prosecuted her on the reservation. It is of note that she does not have an official address as the cabin is in the national forest. The house does not have running water or a septic system. Personal care is completed in the "outhouse." Laundry is done at the local laundromat when there is money for laundry. There is a hand pump to obtain water that can be heated for bathing.

Robert grew up in the "woods." He and his friends played and raised each other until they were school age. Because his family was well-known for selling wood in the community, it was apparent to the teachers when he did not attend school. He was frequently labeled as a truant.

Part of the reason he did not want to attend school was that the other kids made fun of his long hair, second-hand clothing that was frequently dirty and torn, and his lack of academic ability. He was, however, an outstanding athlete in wrestling and basketball. Physically he was solid due to his physical work with his family. He loved basketball and built a hoop that he could throw logs through.

Because he was classified as truant and breaking laws on tribal land, he was entered into the Tribal Juvenile Justice System present in the Northern region. There are 574 federally recognized tribes in the United States.[1] Each of these tribes is a separate sovereign nation in the United States, entirely different from state governmental structures. Each nation has the power to create laws that are separate from those of the state and federal governments. Consequently, they can prosecute people who break those laws on their lands[2]. Robert clashed with both local officials and tribal officials as a young child by being truant and as an older child by fighting, stealing, and being insubordinate on tribal lands.

The juvenile justice system tends to re-traumatize rather than heal.[3] Because of his history of fighting, stealing, and truancy, Robert was removed from his home and placed in a juvenile detention center. At age 12, although he did not understand why he had to "go to jail" and his mother did not, he was at least able to be clean, have regular meals, and begin learning about his history.

Robert's history is significant for multiple adverse childhood events. He was born in poverty to a single-mother household and frequently had no one to protect him; his mother has a history of substance and alcohol use and abuse. Robert does not admit to having been verbally or physically abused; however, he felt that being slapped or beat happens to everyone and is not unusual. He lost his identity as a Native American due to his grandparents' denial of their heritage.

Vulnerabilities

In this situation, the deficits in health care include:

1. Access to tribal health care centers due to his "non-Native" status
2. Health care access in a rural area
3. Behavioral health inpatient care within a reasonable distance, lack of available beds
4. Education was patchy due to his lack of attendance, and he did not finish high school
5. Intermittent detainment in a juvenile detention center
6. Lack of community support
7. Lack of family support
8. Lack of traditional understanding of cultural norms and subtleties
9. Inadequate mentoring
10. Because of his genetic heritage, he has strong Native American physical characteristics (discrimination).

By not acknowledging his Native heritage, Robert is not eligible for health care administered through the Bureau of Indian Affairs. In this state, there are no inpatient hospitals for Native Americans (**Fig. 1**).

This map identifies Indian Health Centers and hospitals in the United States. In this state, there are no IHS facilities. There are 12 tribal health centers, with 6 in the upper region and 6 in the lower area of the state. These tribal centers offer various services depending on their relationships with rural health centers. Some services such as substance use and treatment, primary care, pharmacy, and dentistry are provided by "contract services" contracted through the state and not necessarily supported by the Indian Health Service (IHS).

According to their Web site,[5] the IHS is responsible for providing health care services to Native Americans and Alaska Natives. It is a part of the US Department of Health and Human Services, a cabinet-level position. The service was begun in 1787 due to government-to-government treaties and laws. The IHS provides a "comprehensive health delivery system" for American Indians and Alaska Natives. Access to care is limited by the lack of services in Michigan and other areas of the United States. There are 26 IHS hospitals in the United States. However, to access these services, one must present a tribal membership card or Certificate of Indian Blood (CDIB). The CDIB does not ensure tribal enrollment and thus access to care. Each tribe has its own registration rules. Generally, a person must prove their relationship to an ancestor recorded on the rolls of Native Americans.

In some states, the willingness and ability to enroll in a tribe is financially based, and many tribes have stringent criteria for enrollment. After multiple breaches of treaties and historical abuse and maltreatment, many native/indigenous people avoid contact with the US Government and bureau of indian affairs (BIA).

At this point, the social determinants of health (SDOH)[6] affecting Robert include

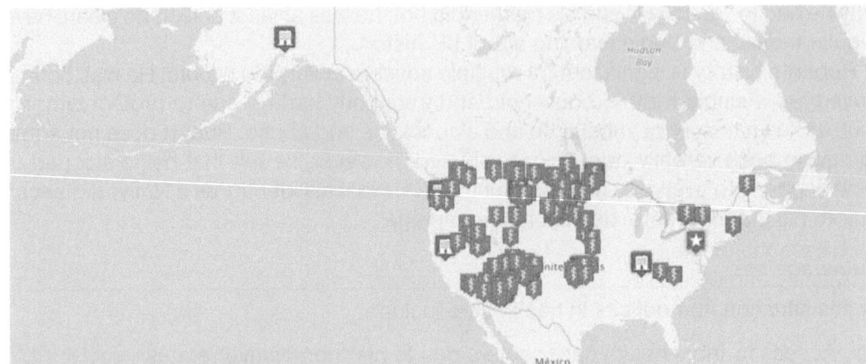

Fig. 1. The Indian Health Service (IHS) is divided into 12 physical areas in the United States: Alaska, Albuquerque, Billings, California, Great Plains, Nashville, Navajo, Nashville, Oklahoma, Phoenix, Portland, and Tucson. Note that there are large geographic areas without specified IHS facilities. OpenStreetMap is *open data*, licensed under the Open Data Commons Open Database License by the OpenStreetMap Foundation. (*Source*: "OpenStreetMap contributors."[4])

1. Economic insecurity
2. Lack of formal education
3. Lack of access to health care
4. High rate of violence
5. Unsafe drinking water
6. Lack of hygiene facilities
7. Lack of community and family support.

INTERSECTIONALITY WITH POVERTY AND GEOGRAPHIC LOCATION

Generational poverty is defined as a family living in poverty for at least two generations.[7] Poverty is not just lacking financial resources to meet basic living requirements. It is also about lack of education, parenting, and spiritual emptiness that create hopelessness.[7] People caught in generational poverty have values centered more on survival and short-term outcomes. Although Robert works, he does not have or value education; he lives his life day to day, often scrambling to get essential resources. He does not have an address as the family home is on state forest property. He has been "told" that he cannot access services and safety nets for the poor. He is eligible for Medicaid; however, he has been unable to find a provider willing to treat his substance use effectively and prefers to continue to use. He feels hopeless over his situation.

Robert lives in a rural part of a northern state. The complicating factors associated with living in a rural area include:

1. Distance to tertiary care. Robert is 100 miles away from an inpatient treatment facility. He does not have a car; no emergency medical service (EMS) is available to transport him. The rural access hospital does not offer psychiatric services.
2. Ability to access primary care services. The average wait time to access primary care is 2 months. One must apply to become a patient. At least four primary care providers (PCPs) have retired or left the area in the past 5 years. Recruiting providers is difficult. Loan forgiveness is helpful. However, these providers go as soon as their loans are paid.

3. Lack of access to fresh fruits and vegetables. Most foods are prepared and contain high levels of fat and salt. Food banks and other commodity programs provide processed food. A disruption of connection to his heritage also results in disconnection from native foodways.
4. Lack of access to education. general educational development (GED) programs are limited in rural school districts.
5. Broadband is scattered throughout the area. Internet in the forest does not exist.
6. Drug use disorders are multifactorial. Socioeconomic and limited education increase the risk of drug use disorders and worsen their consequences.[8]
7. Making and selling drugs are more lucrative than small machine shops or the tourist industry in rural areas.

SUMMARY

Robert is a young man with a difficult life and minimal resources due to generational challenges, such as the intentional destruction of native communities and cultures. If not addressed, he also has multiple social determinant deficiencies that will continue to plague his life and health status. Because he was using an illegal substance and taken to the hospital, he was placed in the county jail on drug charges. Consequently, he could not raise bail and remained in custody, where he caught COVID-19. Fortunately, he survived; however, he needs follow-up treatment for his many challenges. In the health care system, care needs are often not addressed because of a lack of attention to a person's determinants of health. There may not be a pharmacy, a hospital or primary care clinic, a grocery store, exercise facilities, counseling, and other services in the rural area. The nurse then becomes a critical resource in these communities, and it is up to the nurse to know and understand what is achievable and what is not in the plan of care.

CLINICS CARE POINTS

- Robert's needs seem overwhelming.
- Acceptance of his value as a human being is critical.
- Positive regard for him as a patient will build a therapeutic environment.
- Referral to agencies within the community such as community mental health, rural health clinic, and Department of Health and Human Services needs to be made.
- Exploration of his race status needs to occur to secure mentorship, a sense of belonging, and an understanding of the cultural norms of being part of a tribe.[9]
- Offering treatment centers that use traditional healers as part of the care team is effective.[10]
- Medically, Robert must be enrolled in a comprehensive substance use/abuse clinic that can prescribe suboxone and other medications known to treat addiction.
- Reaching out to Native communities with different resources and abilities to enroll him in a tribe.
- Reaching out to his family to identify why it is essential that he become aware of his community and community resources.
  - Many tribes have drum circles with many rigid rules of behavior but are also taught by tribal elders.
  - Many tribes have singers, a traditional ceremonial function to help build a sense of belonging and provide ceremonies for the tribes and surrounding areas.
- Make sure he carries Narcan 4 mg nasal spray.

- Assign a psych mental health nurse practitioner (NP) to coordinate substance use care who understands the native culture, preferably an NP who is Native American.
- Investigate jobs that may accept recreational use of marijuana but no other drugs. Marijuana use is legal in this particular state.
- Provide financial bridge until employed.
- Use a mentoring relationship to facilitate moving through systems.

IMPLICATIONS FOR NURSING EDUCATION TO BUILD RESILIENCE

Several studies have demonstrated that a culturally competent nursing workforce improves health outcomes.[11] Currently, only 0.4% of nurses nationwide identify as American Indian/Alaska Native.[11] Recruitment of nurses from diverse communities can help provide culturally competent care by practitioners who reflect the diversity of the populations they see. McFarland and Wehbe-Alamah present the need for Cultural Care Theory to guide translational research projects, develop appropriate policies and procedures, and promote marketing for and to nursing students from rural, underserved, and diverse backgrounds.[12] With technology, simulation, and innovative service-learning programs, educational needs can be assessed, and innovative curricula developed.

POLICY

Health policy is crucial to providing equitable treatment for people of color and rural communities. Larger health care systems may have a presence in a rural community but only as a critical access facility. Financial constraints and lack of reliable transportation are significant barriers for many. A lack of paid time off, health insurance, childcare, or backup caregivers for vulnerable family members can be insurmountable obstacles for some in rural areas and communities of color.

Nurses are the most numerous health care providers, with 4.2 million nurses in the United States as of 2021.[11] Nurses are also seen as the most ethical, trusted, and honest health care providers for the nineteenth year in a row.[13] Consequently, nurses need to be used in policy decisions by communities, states, and federal levels. Nurses on Boards is an initiative by the American Nurses Association to have nurses' voices heard in the policy-making arena of business and legislation.

Nurses need to become involved in their communities and lobby for underserved populations. Each school system needs to consider the number of school nurses necessary to help identify children at risk for negative social determinants of health (SDOH). The use of Federally Qualified Health Centers and Rural Health Clinics is effective models for providing primary care. However, not enough Physicians, Nurse Practitioners, and Physician Assistants are available to staff these highly effective clinics. Each clinic should reflect the community it serves and build appropriate interventions accordingly. Nurses on community boards and boards of the clinics will help identify interventions that would be effective as they work and live in the community.

Community/University/Communitycollege partnerships assist community economic development. Students who are poor or attend schools in rural areas are not highly recruited for the university setting. Community colleges can be critical access points for training in rural areas. Higher education institutions need to invest in communities to advocate for infrastructure like universal broadband access to connect rural and underserved communities.

Nutrition in rural communities is a challenge. Many rural areas are food deserts, and people are at the mercy of supply chains. Healthy foods such as fruits and vegetables can be accessible using personal and community gardens. Traditional food preservation can be taught through community education programs and school-based efforts.

All these efforts are in process in one way or another, in one community or another, but the steps need to be ramped up. Emphasis on gainful employment, traditional foods and ceremonies, and community infrastructure is critical to helping people like Robert grow and thrive in a rural or indigenous community. Nurses can make these goals happen.

DISCLOSURE

The author has no conflicts of interest or commercial interests associated with this article.

REFERENCES

1. Indian Entities Recognized and Eligible to Receive Services from the United States Bureau of Indian Affairs; Correction AGENCY: Bureau of Indian Affairs, Interior. Federal Register/Vol. 86, No. 67/Friday, April 9, 2021/Notices. Available at: https://www.federalregister.gov/documents/2021/01/29/2021-01606/indian-entities-recognized-by-and-eligible-to-receive-services-from-the-united-states-bureau-of. Accessed January 04, 2022.
2. National Congress of American Indians. Tribal Juvenile Justice: Background and recommendations. 2019. Available at: https://www.ncai.org/resources/ncai_publications/tribal-juvenile-justice-background-recommendations. Accessed January 15, 2022.
3. United States Department of Health and Human Services, Prevention Institute A community approach to address health disparities. Available at: https://minorityhealth.hhs.gov/assets/pdf/checked/thrive_finalprojectreport_093004.pdf. Accessed January 15, 2022.
4. OpenStreetMap® is *open data*, licensed under the Open Data Commons Open Database License (ODbL) by the OpenStreetMap Foundation (OSMF). Available at: https://www.ihs.gov/locations/#:~:text=The%20Indian%20Health%20Service%20is,day%2Dto%2Dday%20basis. Accessed January 15, 2022.
5. Indian Health Services. IHS.gov/overview (N.D.).
6. U.S Department of Health and Human Services, Office of Disease Prevention and Health Promotion (n.d.). Available at: https://health.gov/healthypeople/objectives-and-data/social-determinants-health. Accessed January 2 2022.
7. Urban Ventures. (n.d.). Available at: https://urbanventures.org/facts-about-poverty. Accessed 2 January 2022.
8. Saenz E, Gerra G, Busse A, et al. United Nations Office on Drugs and Crime (UNODC), Austria. Socioeconomic inequalities and drug use disorders: Current knowledge and future directions for research and action. National Institute on Drug Abuse. 2020. Available at: https://www.drugabuse.gov/international/abstracts/socioeconomic-inequalities-drug-use-disorders-current-knowledge-future-directions-research-action. Accessed January 4, 2022.
9. American Association of Colleges of Nursing. The voice of academic nursing. Fact Sheet: Enhancing diversity in the nursing workforce. 2019. Available at: https://www.aacnnursing.org/Portals/42/News/Factsheets/Enhancing-Diversity-Factsheet.pdf.

10. Akridge S. 2020. Available at: https://khn.org/news/reversing-history-indian-health-service-seeks-traditional-healers/. Accessed January 24, 2022.
11. The University of St. Augustine for Health Sciences. Sixty key nursing statistics and trends for 2021. 2021. Available at: https://www.usa.edu/blog/nursing-statistics. Accessed January 2, 2022.
12. McFarland MR, Wehbe-Alamah HB. Leininger's theory of culture care diversity and universality: An overview with a historical retrospective and a view toward the future. J Transcult Nurs 2019;30(6). https://doi.org/10.1177/1043659619867134.
13. Gaines K. Nurses.org. Nurses have been ranked the most trusted profession for 19 years. 2021. Available at: https://nurse.org/articles/nursing-ranked-most-honest-profession/. Accessed January 7, 2022.

Applying Cultural Intelligence to Improve Vaccine Hesitancy Among Black, Indigenous, and People of Color

Angela Richard-Eaglin, DNP, MSN, FNP-BC, CNE, FAANP[a,*],
Michael L. McFarland, DNP, AGACNP-BC, FNP-BC[b]

KEYWORDS

- Cultural intelligence • Mindfulness • Vaccine hesitancy • Structural racism
- COVID-19

KEY POINTS

- With the COVID-19 virus being a novel disease with scientific discovery occurring in real time, trust and reluctance is magnified.
- Structural racism and unethical research practices have contributed to resistance to COVID-19 vaccines and treatments among Black, Indigenous, and People of Color (BIPOC).
- Cultural intelligence can contribute to clinician's understanding of cultural beliefs and practices that may impact vaccine reluctance.
- Cultural intelligence, emotional intelligence, and mindfulness can facilitate trust building among clinicians and patients to improve openness to the COVID-19 vaccine.

INTRODUCTION

There is much criticism surrounding resistance to the COVID-19 vaccine. The problem is that not much thought is given to the possible reasons behind the vaccine resistance and hesitancy. According to the World Health Organization Strategic Advisory Group of Experts on Immunization, vaccine hesitancy is defined as the delay in acceptance or refusal of vaccines despite the availability of vaccination services.[1] Despite the overwhelming evidence to support the benefits of vaccines for preventable diseases and improving health outcomes throughout the world, vaccine hesitancy has been around for centuries.[2] Growing concerns over vaccine hesitancy, resistance, and reluctance were already present before the COVID-19 pandemic.[3] With the COVID-19 being a novel disease with scientific discovery occurring in real time, trust and reluctance

[a] Yale School of Nursing, PO Box 27399, West Haven, CT 06477, USA; [b] Emory University, Nell Hodgson Woodruff School of Nursing, 1520 Clifton Road, Atlanta, GA 30322, USA
* Corresponding author.
E-mail address: angela.richard-eaglin@yale.edu

Nurs Clin N Am 57 (2022) 421–431
https://doi.org/10.1016/j.cnur.2022.04.008

are magnified. It is difficult for nonscientists to grasp the idea that frequent updates in information as new insights are gained contribute to mistrust and increased reluctance to participate in prevention and treatment measures. Vaccine hesitancy perpetuates disease progression and deaths. Among Black, Indigenous, and People of Color (BIPOC) the pervasiveness of inequities in resource availability and other discriminatory practices that created the social determinants of health and proliferated health disparities directly impacted the number of infections and deaths reported in marginalized communities since the outbreak of the COVID-19 pandemic.[4]

The world has been dealing with the COVID-19 pandemic for more than 2 years now. As of March 2021, there have been more than 114.5 million recorded global cases of COVID-19 and 2.54 million COVID-19 related global deaths.[5] In the United States alone, more than 30 million people have been diagnosed with COVID-19, with more than 590,000 deaths as of June 2020.[6] These alarming statistics validate the significant need for prevention through medical intervention.

Further exploration of the statistics reveals that BIPOC has suffered tremendously and disproportionately from COVID-19. According to Laurencin, BIPOC accounts for 1 in 800 COVID-19 deaths nationally, whereas White Americans account for 1 in 3125 COVID-19 deaths.[4] Mortality from COVID-19 for BIPOC is 2.7 times higher than Whites. Black Americans account for 13.4% of the US population and 24% of COVID-19 deaths.[7] Based on statistical data associated with COVID-19-related health outcomes for Black and other marginalized communities of color, one could surmise that in similar circumstances in which new pathogens invade society, the outcomes could be similar. This validates the reality of the impact of structural racism on health disparities and increased morbidity and mortality among BIPOC and emphasizes the need to develop strategic actions that advance health equity. Despite having a 10% higher risk of contracting COVID-19, being 3 times more likely to be hospitalized from coronavirus infection, and having a 2 times higher risk of death, hesitancy and resistance to vaccination continue to persist among BIPOC.[8]

It is essential that health-care providers explore historical and cultural suppositions surrounding BIPOC beliefs and opinions regarding participation in newly developed medical advances. Critical and deliberate consideration must be given to historical factors that continue to perpetuate mistrust in the health-care system. This article will explore vaccine hesitancy and apprehension through a cultural intelligence (CQ) lens and outline possible contributing factors through a historical context. It will also provide some recommended strategies that nurses can apply to clinical practice.

BACKGROUND

People from historically marginalized and oppressed populations continue to suffer from generational trauma associated with structurally racist and oppressive systems that impact all aspects of health. Transformation of these systems in health care implores nurses and other health-care providers to consciously consider that reality. Strategic planning for increasing COVID-19 vaccine participation among BIPOC requires acknowledgment and consideration of cultural and historical variables. The complicated nature of scientific discovery in real time compounded by the historical influence of unethical and inhumane health-care research and clinical practices contributed to resistance and failure of BIPOC to seamlessly engage in obtaining the vaccine. Establishing trusting relationships with BIPOC is a key element for nurses to consider in impacting education and buy-in related to the coronavirus and the COVID-19 vaccine. It also important to note that there are many nuanced cultural differences and causal factors that are vital to consider in provider–patient relationship building.

Controversies

Structural racism is defined as a system resulting from institutional policies and practices that reinforce racial inequities.[9] Systems and institutional frameworks predicated by centralization of Whiteness in ways of being, doing, thinking as the norm or standard spawned foundational layers (**Fig. 1**) that have historically ignored or diminished the health needs of non-White populations. Unfortunately, this failure to consider multiple lived experiences, cultures, and ways of existing created a distortion in the perception of the "why," "what," and "how" in terms of refusal or hesitancy in vaccine reception. "Why" are people from BIPOC and other marginalized communities skeptical and mistrusting of medicine and science? "What" are the precipitating factors? "How" do cultural beliefs impact decisions? These are all questions that clinicians should consider before labeling or judging people whose beliefs and decisions differ from theirs. The alarming realities of the impact of coronavirus on BIPOC have compelled scientists and clinicians to focus at disparities and acknowledge the contribution of racism to inequitable health outcomes. The Centers for Disease Control and Prevention, National Institutes of Health, and other national funding agencies have prioritized investigations and initiatives aimed at examining the connections among structural racism, health disparities, research participation, and vaccine hesitancy.

Inequitable systems, unethical research studies, and medical practices are direct contributors to mistrust and hesitancy related to science and health care among BIPOC. It is imperative that clinicians acknowledge the historical perspectives when soliciting vaccine participation. The *Tuskegee Study of Untreated Syphilis in the Negro Male* is one contributor of reluctance and fear.[10] This was an observational United States Public Health Services study conducted on Black men in Tuskegee, Alabama, for 40 years.[10] The study initially involved 600 Black men, of whom 399 were infected with syphilis, and none were allowed the opportunity to give informed consent.[10] Researchers did not tell the men the truth about the purpose of the study, and participants were not offered or provided with treatment once it became available.[10] Under the guise of incentive for participation in the study, the men received free medical examinations, free meals, and burial insurance.[10]

Another instance in which structural racism was a contributing factor to mistrust and hesitancy to participate in scientific discovery is the unethical, unconsented research

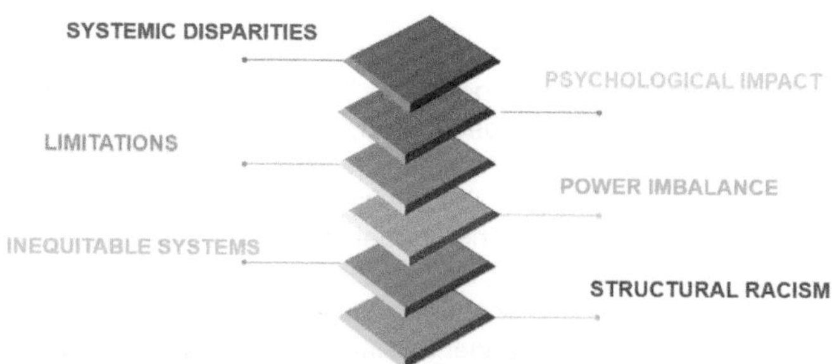

Fig. 1. Multiple variables or layers have historically impacted and continue to influence mistrust of the health-care system among BIPOC. Structural racism is the foundation that created inequitable systems, power imbalances, limitations, negative psychological repercussions, and ultimately, systemic health disparities. Each layer must be considered in isolation and in totality to understand the prevailing issues surrounding vaccine hesitancy.

and subsequent deception and profiting from Henrietta Lacks' appropriately named "immortal cells."[11,12] Henrietta Lacks was a young, impoverished Black woman whose cervical cancer cells were shared with researchers without her knowledge or consent.[11,12] Although Ms. Lacks gave informed consent for surgery related to her cancer, she did not give consent to collect and share her tissue specimens for research.[11] Biomedical researchers named her cells HeLa, using the first 2 initials of her first and last name.[11,12] HeLa cells have been used in pioneered notable research efforts that contributed to the development of the polio vaccine, cloning, gene mapping, in vitro fertilization and much more. Her cells were mass-produced and sold for profit, whereas she and her family lived in poverty.[12] These cells are still being used for extant research and treatment developments. This is a prime example of the historical and structural lack of regard for and exploitation of people from marginalized populations. It is important to note that the Tuskegee study and the Henrietta Lacks situation contributed to the development of ethical research principles and laws.

Power imbalances created by limited representation of BIPOC providers limit influence, increase vulnerability, have a negative psychological impact, and perpetuate structural racism and its corollaries. Structural racism and power imbalances create additional limitations and further disadvantages for historically underrepresented, marginalized, and stigmatized populations. This domino effect was quite evident in the outset of the coronavirus pandemic when access to testing was scarce for people from underrepresented and underserved populations.

Nurses must be aware of the negative psychological impact that marginalization has on people who experience it. People often feel devalued and choose not to access or consistently participate in health care. This consequently inhibits progress and negatively impacts health outcomes. Systemic disparities are a result of biased, incongruent interactions with and inconsistencies in approaches to health care for BIPOC and other individuals from marginalized and stigmatized groups. Marginalization affects all aspects of personhood, including physical, mental, social, and environmental health.[13,14] Hall and colleagues[14] defined marginalized as peripheralization of people based on identities, affiliations, experiences, and environment. Hesitancy and refusal to get the COVID-19 vaccine propagates further marginalization of Black and other people of color because criticism of their choices as irresponsible is made without considering the context within which these decisions are being made.

PERSPECTIVE MATTERS

Cognitive behavior theory suggests that behaviors are largely determined by individual perceptions of the world and lived experiences.[15,16] The adaptive behavioral components (ABC) Model (**Fig. 2**A, B) has been used widely in cognitive behavior therapy, and these concepts can be applied to help clinicians understand individual perceptions about vaccines and other health-care resources that may not be voluntarily accessed by BIPOC communities. This model is explained by 3 factors, the "activating" event, the person's "beliefs" and assumptions about the activating event, and the "consequences" and reactions that result from those beliefs.[22] Understanding how cultural influences and lived experiences influence decisions can assist in navigation of partnerships with individuals, families, and communities who are seeking health-care advice during health-care visits. This insight can inform the clinical approach to educating and interacting with people who are hesitant not only to engage in COVID-19 vaccine reception but also when people from marginalized groups are reluctant to engage in any other medical intervention.

Behavioral ABC Model: Understanding Vaccine Hesitancy

A

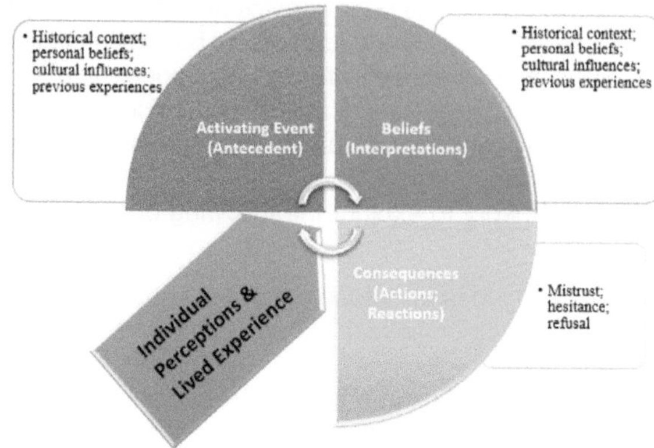

Behavioral ABC Model: Understanding Vaccine Hesitancy

B

A

ANTECEDENT: (Activating Event)

- Historical events
  - Unethical research
  - Racism/bias-influenced care
  - Negative health outcomes
- Preconceptions
- Lived experiences
- Cultural influences

B

BELIEFS (Interpretations)

- Bias
- Racism
- Discrimination
- Negative motives
- Experimentation
- Unethical practices

C

CONSEQUENCES (Actions; Reactions)

- Mistrust
- Hesitance
- Refusal

Fig. 2. (*A*) Antecedents to perception about vaccines include the historical context, personal beliefs, cultural influences, and previous experiences within health-care systems. Interpretations and beliefs are formed because of the same variables from that precede the beliefs: historical context, personal beliefs, cultural influences, and previous experiences. The consequences are the actions and reactions based on the antecedent and the beliefs that are formed from because of the activating event. (*B*) Activating events such as unethical research practices, bias-influenced care, racism, and negative health outcomes for BIPOC people influenced preconceptions about the coronavirus and the COVID-19 vaccine. Lived experiences and cultural influences are also symbiotic with the activating events of historical contexts. Negative beliefs and assumptions about the COVID-19 vaccine are a direct result of fears perpetuated by prolific bias, racism, and discrimination. The beliefs and concerns about negative motives are associated with previous experimentation, unethical research, and substandard health-care practices. The resultant consequences (behaviors/actions/reactions) include mistrust, vaccine hesitance, and vaccine refusal.[17–21]

Attribution theory is also useful in understanding how to build trust and establish healthy relationships with patients who may not be eager to receive vaccines. The broad emphasis of this theory is on assignment of motives to behaviors, both personal and internal, as well as external assignment of motives to others.[17–21] According to attribution theory, after observing behaviors, people opine on whether behaviors are deliberate or not and then ascribe the behaviors to either an intrinsic cause or to a situational cause.[17–21] Motives can be assigned to others based on nonverbal interactions that do not involve direct exchanges and interactions among people.[17–21] Internal motives may be influenced by lived experiences and cultural influences, and external or circumstantial motives may be assigned based on context or contingent on current circumstances and situations.

Clinicians can use this theory to explore the following questions in relation to vaccine hesitancy:

- How do preconceived ideas affect the current situations and interactions?
- How does bias influence interactions with people who are averse to the COVID-19 vaccine?
- How does this affect establishing a trusting relationship?
- What motives are being assigned to the health-care system by BIPOC regarding administration of the COVID-19 vaccine? Why are these motives being assigned? How can I, as a clinician, be an ally for this community?
- How can I effectively support or impact attitudes, behaviors, and opinions among BIPOC communities regarding the COVID-19 vaccine?

Much of how relationships are managed is influenced by individual perceptions of others. Establishing relationships and building trust are essential for effective patient–provider partnerships in health care. Clinicians must be cognizant of personal perspectives and simultaneously attuned with the perspectives of the persons to whom care is delivered. Cultural illiteracy can be detrimental to health outcomes because misinformation and knowledge gaps about cultural differences often catalyze stereotypes and bias. Conversely, cultural literacy and fluency can have a profound effect on openness to differences, understanding opposing preferences and choices, and improving health outcomes for people from underrepresented populations. Through development and application of CQ, clinicians can acquire mindfulness of implicit thoughts that may manifest as visceral reactions and translate to untoward words and behaviors aimed at marginalized individuals. This is important in terms of strategies that lend to mitigating bias-influenced health-care decisions, especially those based on misperceptions and stereotypes.

Application of Cultural Intelligence to Impact Attitudes About Vaccine Hesitancy

Oftentimes, individuals and groups are judged, labeled, and stereotyped because as humans, we see things from personal life experiences and preferences rather than from a global perspective that offers consideration of multiple perspectives. Most clinicians operate from a humanitarian state of mind and embody humanitarian principles. Subsequently, espousing these principles may engender frustrations with people when they forego opportunities to achieve or maintain a so-called healthy state. This frustration may fuel negative clinician attitudes toward people who opt out of obtaining the COVID-19 vaccination.

CQ is a globally recognized, evidence-based approach to assessing and improving effectiveness in culturally diverse interactions.[23] It is defined as the skill and confidence to work effectively in diverse or multicultural situations and environments.[24] Developing and effectively using CQ depends on individual levels of emotional intelligence (EQ). EQ measures perception, management, expression, and evaluation of personal emotions, as well as the ability to interact within interpersonal relationships in prudent and empathetic ways.[25] Cultural and emotional intelligence (EQ) are interdependent and obligatory for establishing and sustaining productive relationships within cross-cultural/multicultural relationships.[23] There are 3 levels of CQ (**Table 1**): low, moderate, and high.[23,24] The level of CQ displayed may vary depending on context and other factors, such as level of EQ, situational distractions, and lack of planning.[23,24]

The CQ framework (**Fig. 3**) has 4 distinct capabilities that, when applied collectively, work together to improve the understanding of different perspectives, enhance effective communication, and ultimately strengthen partnerships and collaborations.[23] In general, consistent application of CQ enhances open-mindedness and facilitates accommodation of different ways of being.[23,24] Clinicians can use CQ to develop conscious awareness of personal feelings, assess knowledge gaps, and gauge readiness to effectively interact with patients from marginalized populations. There is an inherent sense of comfort to interact in the space of sameness and commonalities. Cultural intelligence (CQ) offers opportunities to intentionally learn about cultural differences. Clinicians who with a moderate-to-high CQ can optimize interactions with patients whose beliefs about vaccines or other medical and nursing interventions are incongruent with their own. Additionally, clinicians can use CQ to develop an understanding of where personal biases, attitudes, and perspectives originated, as well as understand and adapt to the cultural differences that contribute to the perspectives, biases, and attitudes of others. Consistent use of CQ during patient interactions has several benefits including but not limited to the following:

- Mindfulness and acceptance of differences and unique lived experiences (ie, unconventional health-care practices, beliefs, attitudes about health and health care)
- Openness to different perspectives
- Development of customized patient visits and treatment plans
- Effective and trusting patient (person), family, and community partnerships
- Greater influence on informed patient (person) decision-making

Additional Strategies and Considerations

Vaccine hesitancy in marginalized communities, particularly the COVID-19 vaccine, poses a crucial challenge to public health on a national and global level. Both empathy and truthful information are essential in reducing hesitancy. Addressing vaccine uptake disparities requires a multipronged strategy that focuses on the needs of marginalized communities. This strategy must acknowledge that vaccine hesitancy is rooted in systemic and structural racism. It should be designed to help BIPOC regain trust in the government and the medical establishment. According to Bogart and colleagues[7], lack of honesty from the government regarding the origins of the pandemic and the vaccine is a leading factor in vaccine hesitancy. Additionally, vaccine hesitancy among BIPOC results from the limited data on the long-term adverse effects of the COVID-19 vaccine.[6] Complete transparency regarding the risks and benefits of vaccines and providing reassurance on robust vaccine safety is necessary to minimize vaccine hesitancy.[26]

Most times, truthful information about vaccines is not enough. BIPOC need culturally sensitive efforts to build trust in the medical information about vaccines discussed in the literature. According to Shen and Dubey, individuals who receive vaccine advice from their family physicians are more likely to trust the information that they are provided.[26] In addition, face-to-face counseling with up-to-date vaccine information from a family physician compared with information gathered from the Internet, family, and friends is received entirely better by marginalized communities.[26]

Table 1
The 3 levels of cultural intelligence: low, moderate, and high[23,24]

Levels of Cultural Intelligence (CQ)		
Low CQ	**Moderate CQ**	**High CQ**
Low CQ is evidenced by the following: • Reacting to external influences during multicultural interactions • Judgements being made about others from personal cultural contexts • Ignoring or marginalizing cultural differences	Moderate CQ is evidenced by the following: • Recognition of other cultural norms and accommodating or adapting into thoughts and behaviors • Interest in learning more about cultural differences but may still focus on commonalities among people	High CQ is evidenced by the following: • Adaptation to other cultural norms as needed • Embracing cultural differences to enhance innovation • Subconscious ability to interrelate in multicultural contexts • Knowledge that homogeneous cultures are not monolithic • Sustained interest in cultural diversity • Ongoing efforts to understand cultural differences • Planning for multicultural interactions, with recognition that each situation is unique • Being flexible in all multicultural interactions

Family physicians who marginalized people trust can soften the mistrust that BIPOC communities have in the medical establishment and pharmaceutical companies, which stems from a history of unethical research practices. Trust can be strengthened if the vaccine information is disseminated by physicians and nurses from the same ethnic background.

Community campaigns on vaccination awareness can be pivotal in decreasing vaccine hesitancy, especially when there are opportunities for people to ask questions in a nonthreatening environment. Campaigns must be planned and implemented effectively. If the campaign is poorly designed and conducted, it could undermine the campaign's intentions. Because faith is an essential pillar of BIPOC communities, faith-based campaigns to mitigate vaccine hesitancy can be promising.[27] Religious and local opinion leaders have the potential to build trust and vaccine advocacy within BIPOC communities.

However, to ensure that the attitudes and beliefs of community leaders are unbiased and shaped by science, community leaders need training and continuing education on vaccine safety to debunk the narrative in BIPOC communities that vaccines are not safe.[28] The US government can support these efforts by awarding financial grants to religious and community leaders to appropriately train individuals for vaccine advocacy. Pastors have earned communities' trust through years of dedicated service. They can be the empathic listener and trusted messenger that health officials can use to ensure that messages about vaccines are received and accepted.[27] Additional trusted messengers may include educators, responsible and reputable social media

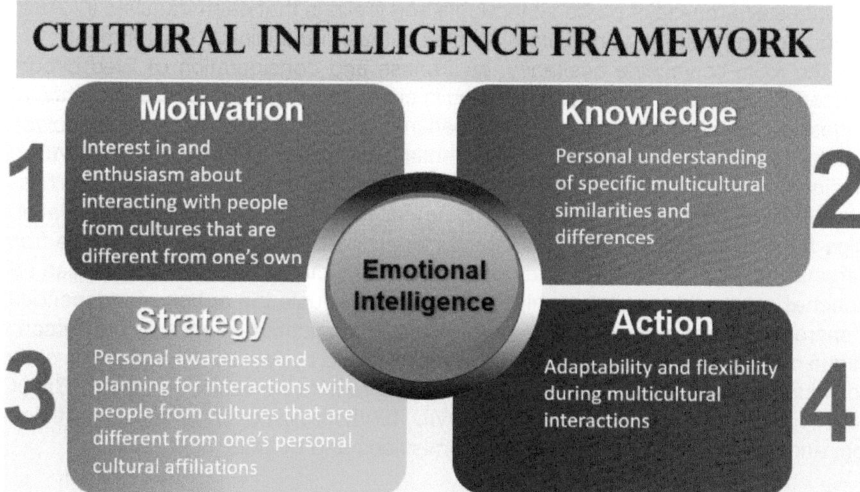

Fig. 3. The CQ framework is composed of 4 distinct capabilities: (1) motivation, (2) knowledge, (3) strategy, and (4) action. During multicultural interactions, application of these 4 functions in tandem with EQ reflects cultural intelligence.[23,24]

platforms, and alternative and complementary medicine practitioners who tend to have a voice during crucial times of vaccine decision-making in BIPOC communities.

CLINICS CARE POINTS

When caring for persons who exhibit vaccine hesitancy or resistance, consider the following:[29]

- Race, ethnicity, nationality, religious affiliations. These characteristics often impact willingness to receive vaccines but do not generalize or make assumptions about individuals based on general demographic categories or cultural practices.
- Conspiracy theories. In a nonthreatening and nonjudgmental manner, probe the person for more information to develop a mutual understanding and dispel any myths about the vaccine.
- Offer evidence-based patient-centered information. If the person refuses, accept it.
- At each clinic visit, offer the vaccine again, unless the patient adamantly states that they are not interested and requests not to engage in the conversation about vaccines at future visits.

SUMMARY

As it relates to opposition to vaccines and other health-care resources, there are times when health-care professionals do not have the time and space to use mindfulness and empathy toward patients/people in the clinical setting. Mindfulness is described as conscious awareness of something.[30] Mindfulness is a technique that can be used to interrupt bias-influenced decisions and actions by assisting people to transfer thoughts from a state of unconscious awareness to a state of conscious awareness. Once thoughts are in the conscious mind, the action that follows can be controlled.[15] Successful use of mindfulness requires time and psychological space to develop conscious awareness of personal thoughts and feelings that often translate into unintended actions that may precipitate sentinel events in the clinical environment.

In the case of vaccine hesitancy, awareness and consideration of lived circumstances of individuals can assist clinicians in circumventing the negative thoughts, attitudes, and behaviors that often impact patient outcomes. Negative behaviors toward people who are vaccine hesitant can potentiate resistance not only to the COVID-19 vaccine but also to mistrusting and accessing the health-care system. Mindfulness, in tandem with EQ and CQ, has a great potential to improve clinician–patient relationships through the development of intentional approaches to caring for people from marginalized populations who may present with reluctance and mistrust. These approaches must include partnerships that offer individuals the option of independent or shared decision-making, provide informed communication specific to the person's unique needs, and consider the lived experiences and current social conditions of the individual. The intended outcome of these strategies is to increase openness of BIPOC individuals to learning more about the COVID-19 vaccine, increase vaccine participation, and decrease COVID-19 hospital admissions and deaths.

DISCLOSURE

The authors do not have commercial or financial conflicts of interests or funding sources.

REFERENCES

1. Liu R, Li GM. Hesitancy in the time of coronavirus: temporal, spatial, and sociodemographic variations in COVID-19 vaccine hesitancy. SSM Popul Health 2021; 15:100896.
2. Siddiqui M, Salmon DA, Omer SB. Epidemiology of vaccine hesitancy in the United States. Hum Vaccin Immunother 2013;9(12):2643–8.
3. Machingaidze S, Wiysonge CS. Understanding COVID-19 vaccine hesitancy. Nat Med 2021;27(8):1338–9.
4. Laurencin CT. Addressing justified vaccine hesitancy in the black community. J Racial Ethnic Health Disparities 2021;8(3):543–6.
5. Jones DL, Salazar AS, Rodriguez VJ, et al. Severe acute respiratory syndrome Coronavirus 2: vaccine hesitancy among underrepresented racial and ethnic groups with HIV in Miami, Florida. Open Forum Infect Dis 2021;8(6):ofab154.
6. Momplaisir FM, Kuter BJ, Ghadimi F, et al. Racial/Ethnic differences in COVID-19 vaccine hesitancy among health care workers in 2 large academic hospitals. JAMA Netw Open 2021;4(8):e2121931.
7. Bogart LM, Ojikutu BO, Tyagi K, et al. COVID-19 related medical mistrust, health impacts, and potential vaccine hesitancy among black Americans living with HIV. J Acquir Immune Defic Syndr 2020;86(2):200–7.
8. Sina-Odunsi AJ. COVID-19 vaccines inequity and hesitancy among African Americans. Clin Epidemiol Glob Health 2021;12:100876.
9. The Aspen Institute. Glossary for understanding the dismantling structural racism/promoting racial equity analysis. In: The aspen institute roundtable on community change. Available at: https://www.aspeninstitute.org/wp-content/uploads/files/content/docs/rcc/RCC-Structural-Racism-Glossary.pdf. Accessed January 17, 2022.
10. The US Public Health Services Syphilis Study at Tuskegee. In: Centers for disease Control and prevention. 2021. Available at: https://www.cdc.gov/tuskegee/timeline.htm. Accessed January 17, 2022.

11. Sodeke SO, Powell LR. Paying tribute to henrietta lacks at tuskegee university and at the virginia henrietta lacks commission, richmond, virginia. J Health Care Poor Underserved 2019;30(4S):1–11.
12. Dimaano C, Spigner C. Teaching from the immortal life of henrietta lacks: student perspectives on health disparities and medical ethics. Health Educ J 2017;76(3): 259–70.
13. Hall JM, Stevens PE, Meleis AI. Marginalization: a guiding concept for valuing diversity in nursing knowledge development. Adv Nurs Sci 1994;16(4):23–41.
14. Hall JM. Marginalization revisited: critical, postmodern, and liberation perspectives. Adv Nurs Sci 1999;22(2):88–102.
15. Beck AT, Rush AJ, Shaw B, et al. Cognitive therapy of depression. New York: Guilford Press; 1979.
16. Yao E, Siegel JT. The influence of perceptions of intentionality and controllability on perceived responsibility. Motiv Sci 2021;7(2):199–206.
17. Penconek T. Theoretical Approaches to studying incivility in nursing education. Int J Nurs Educ Scholarsh 2020;17:20190060.
18. American dictionary of psychology: attribution theory. In: American psychological association. 2020. Available at: https://dictionary.apa.org/attribution-theory. Accessed January 19, 2022.
19. Bardwell R. Attribution theory and behavior change: ideas for nursing settings. J Nurs Educ 1986;25:3122–4.
20. Young SD. The adaptive behavioral components (ABC) model for planning longitudinal behavioral technology-based health interventions: a theoretical framework. J Med Internet Res 2020;22(6):e15563.
21. Zeeman A. ABC model (Albert Ellis). In: Toolshero ABC model of behavior. 2019. Available at: https://www.toolshero.com/psychology/abc-model-albert-ellis/. Accessed January 19, 2022.
22. Lam D, Gale J. Cognitive behaviour therapy: teaching a client the ABC model the first step towards the process of change. J Adv Nurs 2000;31(2):444–51.
23. Livermore D. Cultural intelligence. In: LearnCQ.com. 2022. Available at: https://www.learncq.com/credentials/. Accessed January 20, 2022.
24. Earley PC, Ang S. Cultural intelligence: individual interactions across cultures. Stanford, CA: Stanford University Press; 2003.
25. Salovey P, Mayer JD. Emotional intelligence. Imagination, Cogn Personal 1990; 9(3):185–211.
26. Shen S, Dubey V. Addressing vaccine hesitancy: clinical guidance for primary care physicians working with parents. Can Fam Physician 2019;65(3):175–81.
27. Privor-Dumm L, King T. Community-based strategies to engage pastors can help address vaccine hesitancy and health disparities in black communities. J Health Commun 2020;25(10):827–30.
28. Leask J, Willaby HW, Kaufman J. The big picture in addressing vaccine hesitancy. Hum Vaccin Immunother 2014;10(9):2600–2.
29. Vincen GY, Lasco G, David CC. Fear, mistrust, and vaccine hesitancy: narratives of the dengue vaccine controversy in the Philippines. Vaccine 2021;39(35): 4964–72. https://doi.org/10.1016/j.vaccine.2021.07.051.
30. Khoury B, Knäuper B, Pagnini F, et al. Embodied mindfulness. Mindfulness 2017; 8:1160–71.

Structural Competency in Health Care

Katerina Melino, MS, PMHNP-BC

KEYWORDS

- Structural competency • Structural inequity • Health equity • Health disparities
- Social justice

KEY POINTS

- Structural competency is an evolution of cultural competency, founded on understandings of the social determinants of health and related concepts such as structural violence and structural vulnerability.
- Structural competency offers an alternative framework to the medical model that is strongly aligned with the values of nursing as a profession. This is a powerful position for advocacy and allyship.
- Nurses work with patients who have experienced harms owing to structural violence and vulnerability. The American Nurses Association and Canadian Nurses Association Codes of Ethics require nurses to act on health disparities and work toward social justice.
- Nurses can work to achieve structural competency in clinical practice on the individual, interpersonal, clinic, and community levels.

INTRODUCTION

It has long been recognized that individual health is influenced by factors other than those that are purely biological. The father of "social medicine," Rudolf Virchow, stated more than 200 years ago that health is ultimately a social and political outcome.[1] Over the last 3 decades, there has been a shift in health professions literature in how to consider factors that influence and shape a person's health and health outcomes, from focusing on individual lifestyle choices to acknowledgment and examination of broader factors external to the individual.

The concept of cultural competency in health care was introduced in the 1980s as an important step toward addressing factors that mediate health and the equitable provision of health care.[2] Cultural competency promotes awareness, attitude, and knowledge of other people's cultures in service of improving communication between patients and providers.[3] However, cultural competency over time reduced culture to stereotypes about individuals and groups.[4] It has also been justifiably critiqued on

Psychiatric Mental Health Nurse Practitioner Program, UCSF School of Nursing, 2 Koret Way, Room 511D, San Francisco, CA 94143, USA
E-mail address: katerina.melino@ucsf.edu

Nurs Clin N Am 57 (2022) 433–441
https://doi.org/10.1016/j.cnur.2022.04.009

grounds that someone can never be competent in a culture that is not their own. From this critique arose the idea of cultural humility, which recognizes that one cannot be competent in another culture; rather, it encourages providers to maintain an attitude of continual learning and situating themselves as the nonexpert.[4]

However well-intentioned, both cultural competency and cultural humility fail to change patients' experience of stigma or improve health outcomes because they remain focused at the level of the individual encounter.[5,6,7] In addition, Farmer and colleagues[8] observed that although providers working in clinical care are readily aware of the effect of social and structural determinants on the health of patients, health care providers often lack a formal framework that allows them to apply structural understandings to everyday clinical care.

The framework of structural competency has evolved in response to the significant limitations of cultural competency to fully conceptualize barriers to health faced by patients, and how to address these issues (**Table 1**). Metzl and Hansen[5] define structural competency as follows:

> *The trained ability to discern how a host of issues defined clinically as symptoms, attitudes, or diseases ... also represent the downstream implications of a number of upstream decisions about such matters as health care and food delivery systems zoning laws, urban and rural infrastructures, medicalization, or even about the very definitions of illness and health. (p. 128)*

Scholars suggest that building structural competency is the key to making health care and health systems more equitable, and thus has far-reaching consequences for transforming clinical care and improving patient outcomes.[8] It is important to state that in this context, competency is not synonymous with clinical mastery, as it often is in nursing curricula and clinical evaluation of students. Here, competency refers to the ability to conceptualize the complexity of structures that influence patient health and patient-clinician interactions.[6]

This article describes interventions for working toward structural competency on multiple levels, in the service of improving patient outcomes. Like the US Substance Abuse and Mental Health Administration model of trauma-informed care,[9] achieving structural competency is a multilevel endeavor. This article focuses only on the individual, interpersonal, clinic, and community levels of the framework, as acting on policy and research are outside the purview of immediately actionable interventions.

DEFINITIONS

Clinical Relevance

The literature clearly demonstrates that people facing structural barriers to health and health care owing to institutionalized racism, classism, sexism, homophobia, and ableism, and intersections of these aspects of identity, have significantly higher prevalence of chronically poor health outcomes than those who do not face these barriers.[16–18] The COVID-19 pandemic has starkly reillustrated this reality, both across North America and on a global scale. Statistics show that people of lower socioeconomic status, people of color, and LGBTQ+ people have suffered a disproportionate burden of illness as well as challenges related to the COVID-19 pandemic, such as financial hardship and social isolation.[19,20] The COVID-19 pandemic has occurred in the United States in the context of an already tenuous social safety net and concurrent increase in mental health issues and systemic violence.[21] Even prepandemic, these crises persist when more is known than ever before about the biological impact of social ills on health casts these issues in an even more desperate light.[22] In addition to

Table 1
Definition of structural competency and related concepts

Term	Definition
Structural competency	"The trained ability to discern how a host of issues defined clinically as symptoms, attitudes, or diseases (eg, depression, hypertension, obesity, smoking, medication "noncompliance," trauma, psychosis) also represent the downstream implications of a number of upstream decisions about such matters as health care and food delivery systems, zoning laws, urban and rural infrastructures, medicalization, or even about the very definitions of illness and health"[5]
Structures	"The policies, economic systems, and other institutions (policing and judicial systems, schools, etc) that have produced and maintain social inequities and health disparities, often along the lines of social categories such as race, class, gender, and sexuality"[5]
Structural humility	"The capacity of health care professionals to appreciate that their role is not to surmount oppressive structures but rather to understand knowledge and practice gaps vis-à-vis structures, partner with other stakeholders to fill these gaps, and engage in self-reflection throughout these processes"[11]
Cultural competency	"A set of congruent behaviors, attitudes, and policies that come together in a system, agency, or among professionals that enables effective work in cross-cultural situations"[3]
Cultural humility	"A lifelong process of self-reflection and self-critique whereby the individual not only learns about another's culture, but one starts with an examination of her/his own beliefs and cultural identities"[10]
Social determinants of health	"The physical, environmental, and social conditions in the environments in which people are born, live, learn, work, play, worship, and age that affect a wide range of health, functioning, and quality-of-life outcomes and risks"[12]
Structural violence	"The avoidable impairment of fundamental human needs or…the impairment of human life, which lowers the actual degree to which someone is able to meet their needs below that which would otherwise be possible"[13]
Structural vulnerability	"The outcome of a combination of socioeconomic and demographic attributes (gender, socioeconomic status, race/ethnicity, sexuality, citizenship status, institutional location), in conjunction with assumed or attributed status (including health-related deservingness, normality, credibility, assumed intelligence, imputed honesty)"[14]
Structural racism	"The totality of ways in which societies foster racial discrimination, through mutually reinforcing inequitable systems (in housing, education, employment, earnings, benefits, credit, media, health care, criminal justice, and so on) that in turn reinforce discriminatory beliefs, values, and distribution of resources, which together affect the risk of adverse health outcomes"[15,16]

the COVID-19 pandemic, the last several years of reckoning with systemic racism against black and indigenous peoples across North America, and accelerating climate crises have laid bare the inequities in North American society. Nursing and other health care professions are now critically tasked with examining and responding to health inequities in a different way than before.[23,24] Part of this response must be to recognize and incorporate understandings of factors far outside the individual locus of control that affect health, and act on dismantling such barriers.

RESEARCH

The concept of structural competency is still relatively new in the health care literature, and much of the work on operationalizing this concept relates to doing so in the context of health care professional curricula.[5,6,25,26] However, scholars suggest that structural competency can be the focus of intervention on multiple levels.[21,27–29] Drawing from Neff and colleagues'[27] conceptualization of levels of intervention for structural competency, the remainder of the article summarizes literature that demonstrates structurally competent interventions at the individual, interpersonal, clinic/organizational, and community level. Although policy and research are also crucial levels at which to intervene in working toward structural competency, they represent more long-term solutions that are beyond the scope of this article, which seeks to provide clinical pearls for implementation in practice.

Individual Level: Self-Reflection and Awareness

Scholars define reflection as a "purposeful activity whereby, the individual seeks to look beyond an experience ... towards gaining insight into looking at doing things in a better way, guiding future development."[28] Self-reflection is a foundational aspect of working toward structural competency because the reflective process allows the clinician to recognize what assumptions, values, opinions, and experiences they bring to the clinical encounter, and how these aspects of personal identity consciously, and more often, unconsciously, shape our interactions with clients. Self-reflection allows health care professionals to build awareness of how structures affect them and their clients and subsequently identify ways to assist clients with these barriers.[11] Self-reflection is also emphasized as a component of lifelong learning, which is a professional expectation of nursing.[30] The literature demonstrates that engaging in the process of self-reflection improves communication skills, clinical reasoning skills, and in turn, patient outcomes.[19,31]

The Addressing framework by Hays[32] can be used as a guide to begin the process of critical self-reflection on identity, intersectionality, difference, and power. The Addressing framework facilitates awareness and understanding of the complexities of personal identity in the United States and Canada, including recognition of aspects of socially ascribed identity, such as age, developmental and acquired disabilities, religion, ethnicity, socioeconomic status, sexual orientation, indigenous heritage, national origin, and gender. Addressing offers an exercise whereby the practitioner reflects on each aspect of their identity, and in which aspects they hold power and in which they do not in the context of their lives.[32] This represents the first step in recognizing and understanding how differences in power lead to differences in understandings. It also offers the clinician the opportunity to reflect on the concept of intersectionality in identity as something that must be recognized and negotiated in the provision of clinical care.[33] As a subsequent step, the Addressing framework aids the clinician in thinking through how a patient's multidimensional identity may put them in a position whereby they are more likely to be victims of structural violence and loss of power.

Interpersonal Level: Patient Assessment and Care Planning

Use of an assessment tool to guide clinicians in thinking through social and structural factors that are impacting patients' health can be helpful in starting to build structural awareness. Bourgois and colleagues'[14] Structural Vulnerability Assessment Tool (SVAT) operationalizes structural vulnerability for clinical care delivery by highlighting hierarchical clusters and power relationships that influence individual's health issues. The tool is a 43-item questionnaire that assesses patient needs across 6 domains:

financial stability, physical environment, food security, social support, legal status, and education. It offers a set of questions to ask patients, as well as a set of critical self-reflection questions for the clinician to ask themselves about how they may subconsciously perpetuate structural violence against each patient.[14] It is widely available via an online engine search and has included various repositories of assessment tools validated to assist in measuring health disparities.[34,35] Depending on the clinical setting, the SVAT can also be combined with other screening tools, such as the Barriers to Access to Care Evaluation scale[36] and the Questionnaire on Anticipated Discrimination,[37] to assess patients' internalized stigma related to structural barriers and to capture a picture of what clinic clients are facing overall.[38]

Clinic/Institutional Level: Diverse Hiring and Staff Training

Working toward structural competency at a clinic/institutional level requires organizations to examine how they can foster an understanding of structures affecting health among clinic staff. This includes implementing hiring practices that are holistic and seeking to bring in staff with a wide variety of lived and work experience, and that are attuned to and interested in attending to structural factors as part of clinical care. Another key aspect of structural competency at the clinic level is training opportunities. The training resources available through the Structural Competency Working Group (https://structuralcompetency.org/structural-competency/) are free and available to all; this group is also available for customized consultation and workshop training.[39]

Community Level: Collaboration

At the community level, nurses, staff teams, and clinics can collaborate with community partners to broaden their capability for addressing structural barriers to health. One model of integration that has become increasingly popular in the United States, and demonstrated to contribute to improved patient health outcomes, is the medical-legal partnership (MLP). MLPs are collaborative interventions between health care clinics and community law partners (often nonprofit legal agencies or law schools) that recognize and address the impact of social and environmental factors on health by providing legal remedy.[40] Examples of issues that MLPs work to address include establishing eligibility and accommodations for disability, food stamps, identity-affirming documentation changes, housing rights, eviction assistance, immigration status, domestic violence, family law, and guardianship.[41] In this model, health care lawyers join the interprofessional team on site to provide low-barrier access for clients struggling with these issues.[40] Screening tools, such as the i-HELP, can be used by nurses to identify clients who may need assistance with legal issues and thus facilitate referrals.[41] MLPs are often used to support a particular target population, for example, people living with HIV, immigrants, and/or veterans.[40,42,43] In the United States, the Department of Veterans Affairs and the Health Resources Service Administration support and fund MLPs as tools to improve health equity.[44,45]

DISCUSSION

Incorporating practices of self-reflexive inquiry, assessment tools to identify patients who are at risk for structural violence, clinic-wide training, and collaborative partnerships allows nurses and their organizations to take the first step toward addressing structural barriers at several levels. However, successful implementation of these interventions requires a foundational ability on behalf of health care providers and organizations to have and build capacity for distress tolerance and asking – and answering

– uncomfortable questions. Interventions such as diversifying hiring practices in the name of working toward structural competency are doomed to fail to do so if health care providers, staff, managers, and leaders, both individually and collectively, are not prepared to really listen to and encounter difficult conversations with said new colleagues about how to move forward with change.

Although dismantling structural barriers to health care is neither an easy nor a comfortable endeavor, it is a task we are called to do by our professional mandate as nurses. Structural competency aligns with nursing's mandate for social justice, which is reflected in both the American Nurses Association's (ANA) and the Canadian Nurses Association's (CNA) code of ethics.[46,47] The ANA's code mandates nursing to reduce health disparities and integrate social justice into its work.[46] CNA's code guides nurses to recognize and work to address organizational, social, economic, and political factors that influence health and well-being; recognize and address the social determinants of health; work for social justice; and advocate for change to unhealthy policies.[47] Made explicit, structural competency is implicit in the nursing profession's ethos and mandate across North America.

SUMMARY

Structural competency offers a broad and timely framework through which to consider and act on addressing health inequities. It moves beyond cultural competency and the social determinants of health to situate understandings of health inequity in historical contexts and allow nurses to see how these inequities are continually reproduced in status-quo health care. Structural competency offers an alternative framework to the medical model that is strongly aligned with the values of nursing as a profession. This is a powerful position for advocacy and allyship. Nurses can work to achieve structural competency in clinical practice on the individual, interpersonal, clinic, and community levels.

CLINICS CARE POINTS

Achieving structural competency in health care can take place at the following levels, with examples of appropriate interventions for each level[27]:

- Individual level: critical self-reflection and self-awareness
- Interpersonal level: screening tools to identify and assess clients at risk for structural violence/ vulnerability
- Clinic/organizational level: diversifying hiring practices and workplace training
- Community level: medical-legal partnership collaboration

DISCLOSURE

The author has no commercial or financial conflicts of interest to disclose, nor were any funding sources used to complete this article.

REFERENCES

1. Meili R, Hewett N. Turning Virchow upside down: medicine is politics on a smaller scale. J R Soc Med 2016;109(7):256–8.
2. Henderson S, Horne M, Hills R, et al. Cultural competence in healthcare in the community: a concept analysis. Health Soc Care Community 2018;26(4): 590–603.

3. Substance Abuse and Mental Health Services Administration. Improving cultural competence. Available at: https://store.samhsa.gov/sites/default/files/d7/priv/sma14-4849.pdf. Accessed October 28, 2021.
4. Drevdahl DJ. Culture shifts: from cultural to structural theorizing in nursing. Nurs Res 2018;67(2):146–60.
5. Metzl JM, Hansen H. Structural competency: theorizing a new medical engagement with stigma and inequality. Soc Sci Med 2014;103:126–33.
6. Metzl JM, Hansen H. Structural competency and psychiatry. JAMA Psychiatry 2018;75(2):115–6.
7. Treloar C, Schroeder S, Lafferty L, et al. Structural competency in the post-prison period for people who inject drugs: a qualitative case study. Int J Drug Policy 2021;95:103261.
8. Farmer PE, Nizeye B, Stulac S, et al. Structural violence and clinical medicine. PLoS Med 2006;3(10):e449.
9. Substance Abuse and Mental Health Services Administration. SAMHSA's concept of trauma and guidance for a trauma-informed approach. HHS Publication No. (SMA) 14-4884. Rockville, MD: Substance Abuse and Mental Health Services Administration; 2014.
10. Tervalon M, Murray-García J. Cultural humility versus cultural competence: a critical distinction in defining physician training outcomes in multicultural education. J Health Care Poor Underserved 1998;9(2):117–25.
11. Davis S, O'Brien AM. Let's talk about racism: strategies for building structural competency in nursing. Acad Med 2020;95(12S Addressing Harmful Bias and Eliminating Discrimination in Health Professions Learning Environments):S58–65.
12. Centers for Disease Control [CDC]. Social determinants of health: know what affects health. Available at: https://www.cdc.gov/socialdeterminants/. Accessed October 28, 2021.
13. Galtung J. Violence, peace, and peace research. J Peace Res 1969;6(3):167–91. http://www.jstor.org/stable/422690.
14. Bourgois P, Holmes SM, Sue K, et al. Structural vulnerability: operationalizing the concept to address health disparities in clinical care. Acad Med 2017;92:299–307. https://doi.org/10.1097/acm.0000000000001294.
15. Bailey ZD, Krieger N, Agénor M, et al. Structural racism and health inequities in the USA: evidence and interventions. Lancet 2017;389(10077):1453–63.
16. Kelly BD. Structural violence and schizophrenia. Soc Sci Med 2005;61(3):721–30.
17. Holley LC, Mendoza NS, Del-Colle MM, et al. Heterosexism, racism, and mental illness discrimination: experiences of people with mental health conditions and their families. J Gay Lesbian Soc Serv 2016;28(2):93–116. https://doi.org/10.1080/10538720.2016.1155520.
18. Nazroo JY, Bhui KS, Rhodes J. Where next for understanding race/ethnic inequalities in severe mental illness? Structural, interpersonal and institutional racism. Sociol Health Illn 2020;42(2):262–76.
19. Kim EJ, Marrast L, Conigliaro J. COVID-19: magnifying the effect of health disparities. J Gen Intern Med 2020;35(8):2441–2.
20. Gil RM, Freeman TL, Mathew T, et al. Lesbian, gay, bisexual, transgender, and queer (LGBTQ+) communities and the coronavirus disease 2019 pandemic: a call to break the cycle of structural barriers [published correction appears in J Infect Dis. 2021 Nov 10. J Infect Dis 2021;224(11):1810–20.
21. Hansen H, Braslow J, Rohrbaugh RM. From cultural to structural competency-training psychiatry residents to act on social determinants of health and institutional racism. JAMA Psychiatry 2018;75(2):117–8.

22. Conley D, Malaspina D. Socio-genomics and structural competency. J Bioeth Inq 2016;13(2):193–202.
23. Nardi D, Waite R, Nowak M, et al. Achieving health equity through eradicating structural racism in the United States: a call to action for nursing leadership. J Nurs Scholarsh 2020;52(6):696–704.
24. Scott J, Johnson R, Ibemere S. Addressing health inequities re-illuminated by the COVID-19 pandemic: how can nursing respond? Nurs Forum 2021;56(1):217–21.
25. Woolsey C, Narruhn RA. A pedagogy of social justice for resilient/vulnerable populations: structural competency and bio-power. Public Health Nurs 2018;35(6): 587–97.
26. Waite R, Hassouneh D. Structural competency in mental health nursing: understanding and applying key concepts. Arch Psychiatr Nurs 2021;35(1):73–9.
27. Neff J, Holmes SM, Strong S, et al. The Structural Competency Working Group: lessons from iterative, interdisciplinary development of a structural competency training module. In: Hansen H, Metzl JM, editors. Structural competency in mental health and medicine: a case-based approach to treating the social determinants of health. Cham: Springer International Publishing; 2019. p. 53–74.
28. Hansen H, Metzl J. Structural competency in the U.S. healthcare crisis: putting social and policy interventions into clinical practice. J Bioeth Inq 2016;13(2): 179–83.
29. Graham MM, Johns C. Becoming student kind: a nurse educator's reflexive narrative inquiry. Nurse Educ Pract 2019;39:111–6.
30. Davis L, Taylor H, Reyes H. Lifelong learning in nursing: a Delphi study. Nurse Educ Today 2014;34(3):441–5.
31. Pangh B, Jouybari L, Vakili MA, et al. The effect of reflection on nurse-patient communication skills in emergency medical centers. J Caring Sci 2019;8(2): 75–81.
32. Hays PA. The new reality: diversity and complexity. In: Hays PA, editor. Addressing cultural complexities in practice: Assessment, diagnosis, and therapy. American Psychological Association; 2016. https://doi.org/10.1037/14801-001.
33. Crenshaw K. Demarginalizing the intersection of race and sex: a Black feminist critique of antidiscrimination doctrine, feminist theory and antiracist policies. Univ Chic Leg Forum 1989;1:139–67.
34. University of California San Francisco Social Interventions Research & Evaluation Network. Structural vulnerability assessment tool. Available at: https://sirenetwork.ucsf.edu/tools-resources/resources/structural-vulnerability-assessment-tool. Accessed November 8, 2021.
35. Kaiser Permanente. Systematic review of social screening tools. Available at: https://sdh-tools-review.kpwashingtonresearch.org/. Accessed November 8, 2021.
36. Clement S, Brohan E, Jeffery D, et al. Development and psychometric properties of the Barriers to Access to Care Evaluation scale (BACE) related to people with mental ill health. BMC Psychiatry 2012;12:36.
37. Gabbidon J, Brohan E, Clement S, et al, MIRIAD Study Group. The development and validation of the Questionnaire on Anticipated Discrimination (QUAD). BMC Psychiatry 2013;13:297.
38. Jegede O, Muvvala S, Katehis E, et al. Perceived barriers to access care, anticipated discrimination and structural vulnerability among African Americans with substance use disorders. Int J Soc Psychiatry 2021;67(2):136–43.
39. Structural Competency Working Group. Available at: https://structuralcompetency.org/structural-competency/. Accessed November 8, 2021.

40. Regenstein M, Trott J, Williamson A, et al. Addressing social determinants of health through medical-legal partnerships. Health Aff (Millwood) 2018;37(3): 378–85.
41. National Center for Medical-Legal Partnership. Available at: https://medical-legalpartnership.org/. Accessed November 5, 2021.
42. League A, Donato KM, Sheth N, et al. A systematic review of medical-legal partnerships serving immigrant communities in the United States. J Immigr Minor Health 2021;23(1):163–74.
43. Fuller SM, Steward WT, Martinez O, et al. Medical-legal partnerships to support continuity of care for immigrants impacted by HIV: lessons learned from California. J Immigr Minor Health 2020;22(1):212–5.
44. United States Department of Veterans Affairs. National center for healthcare advancement and partnerships. Available at: https://www.va.gov/healthpartnerships/updates/mlp/mlpadditionalresources.asp. Accessed November 10, 2021.
45. Health Resources and Services Administration. Available at: https://bphc.hrsa.gov/qualityimprovement/strategicpartnerships/ncapca/natlagreement.html. Accessed November 10, 2021.
46. American Nurses Association. Code of ethics for nurses. Available at: https://www.nursingworld.org/coe-view-only. Accessed November 12, 2021.
47. Canadian Nurses Association. Code of ethics for registered nurses in Canada. Available at: https://www.cna-aiic.ca/~/media/cna/page-content/pdf-en/code-of-ethics-2017-edition-secure-interactive. Accessed November 12, 2021.

Considerations and Recommendations for Care of Black Pregnant Patients During COVID-19

Jacquelyn McMillian-Bohler, PhD, CNM, CNE*,
Lacrecia M. Bell, MSN, RN

KEYWORDS

- Black maternal morbidity and mortality • COVID-19 and pregnancy
- Health disparities

KEY POINTS

- Black pregnant patients experience increased rates of morbidity, mortality, preterm labor, depression, and hypertensive disorders in pregnancy.
- Disparities in Black maternal perinatal outcomes persist owing to systemic racism and discrimination and bias within the health care system.
- COVID-19 has exacerbated health disparities among marginalized and vulnerable populations, including Black pregnant persons.
- Environmental exposure, multigenerational living status, lack of access to health care, vaccine hesitancy, and inadequate education about SARS-CoV-2 contribute to the increased rates of COVID-19 within the Black community.

INTRODUCTION

On January 9, 2020, the World Health Organization announced suspicions of a flulike virus in Wuhan, China, potentially linked to the coronavirus.[1] As of January 2022, more than 70.2 million Americans have contracted severe acute respiratory syndrome coronavirus 2 (SARS-CoV-2), and more than 800,000 Americans have died of COVID-19.[5] Although the pandemic has affected nearly every community in the United States, Black, Latinx, and indigenous people remain overrepresented in positive cases and death rate reports.[5] Health disparities among the minority populations in the United States predate the devastating effects of COVID-19[3]. However, as explained by Volkan Bozkir, former president of the United Nations General Assembly, “this pandemic has laid bare the existing vulnerabilities facing the most marginalized and disadvantaged groups.”

Duke University School of Nursing, 307 Trent Drive, Durham, NC 37710, USA
* Corresponding author.
E-mail address: jacquelyn.mcmillianbohler@duke.edu

Nurs Clin N Am 57 (2022) 443–452
https://doi.org/10.1016/j.cnur.2022.04.010

Black pregnant patients are a marginalized and disadvantaged population. It is well documented that Black pregnant patients are more likely than patients from other ethnic identities to experience perinatal complications, such as depression, preterm labor, hypertensive disorders, cardiovascular disorders, and postpartum bleeding.[4] The most disturbing statistic is that Black pregnant patients are 3 times more likely to die in childbirth than White patients.[4] Black patients also experience greater incidences of "near-misses," called severe maternal morbidity (SMM).[4] In the case of an SMM, a complication occurs, and the patient nearly dies. One study reported that Black women are 2.1 times more likely to experience an SMM than hite women.[4] These maternal disparities exist regardless of the education and socioeconomic status of the mother. The root of these health disparities is systemic racism, and discrimination and bias within the health care system.[4] Given the disparities in COVID-19-related health outcomes for Black persons and the preexisting health disparities for Black birthing persons, it is essential to explore the impact of COVID-19 on Black pregnant persons.

Education and data about the management of COVID-19 continue to evolve. As a result, information about the impact of COVID-19 on individual populations is also limited. It is, however, possible for health care providers to make changes in their practice that can improve maternal outcomes for Black pregnant patients. The purpose of this article is to describe factors that may contribute to the differences in COVID-19-related health outcomes for Black people and present a list of recommendations for health care providers to integrate into their clinical practice.

THE OVERALL IMPACT OF COVID-19 ON BLACK PEOPLE

Black people make up only 15% of the US population; however, in 2020, they accounted for 25% of the positive COVID-19 tests and 39% of the recorded COVID-19-related deaths.[5,8] As of October 2021, the disparity in death rates for Black people has narrowed to 17% but remains disproportionate to the overall American population. Factors such as vaccine hesitancy, lack of culturally appropriate education about COVID-19, and general medical mistrust have impacted COVID-related health outcomes.[6] In addition, social determinates of health (defined as where one lives, works, plays, and worships) also appear to play a significant role in the increased rates of SARS-CoV-2 exposure and viral transmission.[7]

Increased Risk for Exposure to SARS-CoV-2

Several factors may increase the opportunity for SARS-CoV-2 exposure for Black persons, including occupational exposure and challenges related to protective equipment. First, Black Americans are more likely to work in industries with a high potential for exposure to SARS-CoV-2.[19] These jobs include work within home health care, medical aide services, manufacturing, housekeeping, and retail industries. These jobs are considered essential, yet the workers often report feeling undervalued,5 and protection against COVID-19 exposure is inconsistent. Once exposed to SARS-CoV-2, workers can unintentionally spread the virus to their families. Minority populations are more likely to live in densely populated settings and multigenerational housing. Therefore, occupational exposure can not only impact an entire family but also impact an entire community.

Second, aside from challenges everyone faced obtaining personal protective equipment, using protection against SARS-CoV-2 has not been race-neutral. According to a Pew study taken at the beginning of the pandemic, 42% of Black Americans were concerned about the most basic protection—wearing a mask. In addition, a University of

North Carolina coronavirus project conducted to explore attitudes and behaviors related to the COVID-19 pandemic found that participants viewed Black men wearing a cloth mask as less trustworthy and threatening.[9] With the murder of George Floyd, Ahmad Avery, Brianna Taylor, and countless other victims on the minds of many Black Americans, any hesitancy to participate in a recommendation that may lead to an increase in suspicion is justifiable.

A Legacy of Medical Mistrust

Examples of poor treatment of Black people by the medical community are legion. Black patients often report feeling dismissed or unheard by providers.[10] Even during this pandemic, Black people seeking health care for symptoms of COVID-19 reported feeling ignored and were denied testing.[11] There are reports of providers dismissing complaints by Black patients who eventually passed away owing to complications of the disease. For example, a video of Dr Moore, who died of complications of COVID-19 after sharing her story of being mistreated in the hospital, went viral. This type of media further sews seeds of mistrust within a community, whether wholly accurate or not.

There are also historical events that illustrate the research community's longstanding mistreatment of Black people. In the Tuskegee study, which lasted more than 40 years, researchers did not consent to the Black men participating in a study. The researchers then withheld treatments for syphilis,[12] resulting in permanent disability or death for some participants. This research study did not end until 1972, within the lifetime of today's Black patient population. In the case of Henrietta Lax, researchers collected a sample of her cervical cells without her knowledge or consent. Those cells were later used to cultivate a cell bank for research and genetic studies. Neither Henrietta nor her family was ever compensated. Finally, Dr Marion Sims, the "father of gynecology," performed brutal experiments on Black enslaved bodies without anesthesia. He believed that Black people did not experience pain the same as White people.[5] As the stories of the horrific events circulate within the Black community, commingling with present-day experiences of bias and discrimination, feelings of mistrust may persevere.

A 2020 survey by the Kaiser Family Foundation and ESPN called "The Undefeated" found that "seven out of 10 Black adults still believe that race-based discrimination in health care happens somewhat often, and one in five say they have personally experienced it in the past year."[5] Considering the legacy of discriminatory treatment of Black people in the name of science, it is understandable that when the COVID-19 vaccine became available in December 2020, some Black people may have had doubts about the vaccine's safety and were hesitant to sign up for vaccinations.

Vaccine Hesitancy and Access to Testing

The results of a Pew study collected in 2020 before the availability of the COVID-19 vaccine revealed that although 60% of Americans reported that they would get the vaccine, only 42% of Black people surveyed would do so.[13] Reasons for low participation in COVID-19 vaccinations may be general medical mistrust and concerns about the how the vaccine was created.

Unfortunately, racial disparity in clinical trial participants persisted in the Moderna and Pfizer-BioTech studies as the COVID vaccine was developed. For example, although 12.5% of the US population is Black, only 9% of the participants in both studies was Black.[14] Failure to include a representative sample in clinical trials may negatively impact the confidence that Black people and other people have about the safety and efficacy of the vaccine. In addition, some people were concerned that the vaccine production speed also meant that the vaccine was not well tested, and unanswered questions may have delayed vaccinations. As of May 2022, only 66% of Americans are fully vaccinated.[15,16] Of those vaccinated, it is estimated that only 10% are Black, which is well below the 12% representation in the whole US population.[17] As broad vaccination of the population is a critical factor in ending this pandemic,[13] recognizing and addressing the underlying barriers for vaccine hesitancy are vital.

Testing is another strategy to contain COVID-19; however, access to COVID testing for some Black people is yet another challenge. In some communities, testing is readily available, or if persons have insurance, they can receive testing at a multitude of settings.[18] In other communities, testing may be free, but the lines for testing may be long. For the client with any symptoms of COVID-19, it may be difficult to find a test location that will take a patient.

COVID-19 AND PREGNANCY

Data about the impact of COVID-19 and pregnancy continue to evolve; however, it appears that the susceptibility rates to SARS-CoV-2 during pregnancy mirror the general population. Because SARS-CoV-2 is overrepresented in the general population, however, it is overrepresented in the Black pregnant population.[17] For pregnant persons who contract COVID-19 during pregnancy, rates of pregnancy complications and unfavorable maternal outcomes are increased.[17] Pregnancy complications may include stillbirth, preterm birth, admission to intensive care unit, and ventilatory support,[20] although this finding is inconsistent between studies.[20] What is consistent in the literature is that pregnant patients, like nonpregnant patients, with comorbidities, such as obesity, diabetes, or hypertensive disorders, are at greater risk for poor outcomes[20] should they contract COVID-19 during pregnancy.

Adverse neonatal effects can be associated with maternal SARS-CoV-2 infection.[20] Although the rates of vertical transmission from the birth person to the fetus are reported to be low, transmission may occur.[21] The inflammatory response caused by SARS-CoV-2 may elicit an inflammatory response on the placenta, decreasing maternal-fetal blood flow. More studies are needed to understand fully COVID-19 on a pregnancy. However, it is noteworthy that the risk of a newborn contracting COVID-19 from the birthing person may be significantly reduced when the birthing person wears a mask and practices hand hygiene.[21]

Black pregnant patients reported a higher rate of mental health diagnoses, including anxiety and stress, than White or Latino people[22] during pregnancy. Reasons for the increased anxiety and stress include exposure to racism and discrimination, concerns about the COVID-19 pandemic, and the potential effects of COVID-19 on the fetus. In addition, a high level of anxiety and stress during pregnancy is associated with higher mortality.[23]

Vaccination is the best defense again the SARS-CoV-2 virus; however, pregnant patients have concerns, and it was reported that pregnant and breastfeeding women were less likely than the general population to accept the COVID-19 vaccine.[22] Concern over the impact of the vaccine was often cited as the reason for the hesitation.

RECOMMENDATIONS FOR HEALTH CARE PROVIDERS

With the knowledge that the effects of COVID-19 will continue within the health care system for years to come, the authors offer recommendations (**Table 1**) that may improve the pregnancy, birth, and postpartum experiences for Black birthing persons. Although the recommendations are based on meeting the needs of Black patients,

Table 1
Recommendations and support for black pregnant persons

Recommendation	Rationale	Considerations
Develop an individualized approach to educating clients about COVID-19 Refer patients to community organizations, faith-based organizations, or Black medical communities providing education about the COVID-19 vaccine[24]	Patients have different individual needs and experiences that should be considered when teaching about COVID-19	Information about COVID-19 is widely available on the Internet but may not be culturally appropriate, accurate, or understood by nonmedical persons
Ask about and *listen* to concerns about COVID-19 and the vaccination[17]	It is essential to provide clear, concise information about COVID-19 and transmission risks for vaccinated and unvaccinated[27]	Black women have frequently reported feeling unseen or unheard as they express concerning symptoms to their providers
Discuss the prenatal visit schedule and offer a flexible schedule[28]Make telehealth visits available for patients when patients need to miss or cancel in-person visits. Ask the client has any needed equioment at home, including urine dipstick, a scale, or a blood pressure cuff.[34]	Black women had the lowest completion of prenatal visits compared with Hispanic and White counterparts during COVID-19. When pregnant women do not receive antepartum care, there is a greater risk of poor health outcomes for the birthing person and the fetus	Some birthing Black persons may be working in the service industry, frontline workers, or caring for other family members, including small children.([2]) With the frequent surges of COVID-19, patients may miss appointments owing to at-home care needs related to COVID-19.
Offer the COVID vaccine at each visit, even if the vaccine has been refused in the past[27] Discuss specific concerns about the vaccine if clients are hesitant[25,27]	Given the current low vaccination rates for Black birthing persons, and Black persons living in the United States, it is essential to continue to offer the COVID-19 vaccine[27]	Historical harms to the Black population may have propagated distrust, and patients may be hesitant about the efficacy and safety of the COVID-19 vaccine. The pregnant client may also be concerned about the effect of the vaccine on the fetus[25,27]

(*continued on next page*)

Table 1
(*continued*)

Recommendation	Rationale	Considerations
Screen for postpartum depression[31] When symptoms of anxiety and depression do present, patients should be referred for appropriate psychological services. Once those referrals are made, maternity care providers should follow up with the referral and patient[31]	Given the increased rates of anxiety and depression for Black birthing patients, providers should screen patients for depression early and often and make referrals when needed. Many of the concerns that patients share include worries about the birthing experience, the presence of the designated support person(s), and financial burdens[31]	Before the pandemic, rates of depression in Black birthing persons were increased. The direct and indirect effects of COVID-19 increased Black pregnant patients vulnerable to COVID-19[30]. Often, patients presenting with anxiety and depression fall in the gap of care to obtain psychological services. Black birthing patients need to be frequently screened informally or formally[32]
Perform a comprehensive assessment of risk factors for COVID-19	Preexisting comorbidities, such as diabetes, hypertension, autoimmune disorders, or obesity, increase the risk of severe COVID-19, and Black women are at increased risk for this disease[21]	Patients with preexisting conditions like obesity, diabetes, and hypertension should be counseled about continued health maintenance of preexisting conditions
Offer telehealth and follow-up for missed prenatal visits	Black pregnant clients are at increased risk for poor health outcomes during pregnancy and may need more frequent visits[29]	Consideration should be given for difficulties the client may experience getting to in-person visits. Time away from work, transportation, or lack of childcare may make it challenging to attend visits Internet access may not be reliable; therefore, it is essential to ensure the patient has access before setting up telehealth visits
Actively listen to patients' concerns	Providers must self-educate on the harm that individual patients or families experienced when engaging the health care community. Providers should refrain from shame and bullying and partner with patients to address their concerns and barriers	Black women reported the lowest confidence in their care[21]

(*continued on next page*)

Table 1
(*continued*)

Recommendation	Rationale	Considerations
Encourage prenatal and postpartum doula services[30]	Continuous labor support has been shown to decrease the rate of cesarean birth and increase birth experience satisfaction[33,30]	Data point to the benefit and positive health outcomes when doulas are present for prenatal support, the birth experience, and postpartum care. Maternity care providers can encourage doulas and liaise with Black doulas to refer their patients[30]
Discuss the use of a support person during labor. Providers may recommend connecting with friends and family over zoom or more frequent phone calls[31]	There may be a limitation to the number of support persons allowed on the unit. Lower levels of social support are associated with higher levels of depression and anxiety during pregnancy[31]	Birth outcomes are improved with continuous labor support. Discussing the options beforehand allows the patient to decide who they want present. In some cases, a doula does not count in the visitor count[30]
Encourage breastfeeding[21]	There is no evidence to support that COVID-19 is spread through breastmilk[21]	If the birthing person delays breastfeeding initiation, there may be difficulties in milk production

universal application of these recommendations would likely benefit all pregnant patients during this pandemic and beyond.

SUMMARY

Black people continue to experience a disproportionate burden of COVID-19. Despite the scientific knowledge that herd immunity may eradicate this deadly virus, the Black population remains significantly undervaccinated. Lack of culturally appropriate education and a history of mistreatment by the health care community may contribute to vaccine hesitancy. Black pregnant women are already considered a vulnerable population because of the increased risk of morbidity and mortality in pregnancy impacted to a greater extent during this pandemic. Preexisting morbidities and mortalities and rates of depression, which were disproportionate before COVID-19, are likely more prevalent now. Special considerations and additional screenings are warranted to ensure that this vulnerable population receives adequate and supportive care. Adopting these recommendations may improve perinatally for Black pregnant patients; however, each recommendation should be adopted for care for all pregnant patients long after this pandemic has passed.

CLINICS CARE POINTS

- Maintain flexibility when describing the prenatal visit schedule. If possible, offer telehealth visits to ensure that patients receive adequate care.[28]

- Ask about and listen to patients' concerns about COVID 19, the vaccine, and the pregnancy.Offer COVID vaccine at each visit even if it has been refused in the past.[20]
- Screen for postpartum depression and follow up with the referral AND the patient.[26]
- Encourage prenatal and postpartum doula services.[31]
- Discuss ongoing support from family and friends during the pregnancy and labor.[32]

DISCLOSURE

The authors have no commercial or funding conflicts to disclose.

REFERENCES

1. WHO statement regarding cluster of pneumonia cases in Wuhan, China. 2020. Available at: https://www.who.int/china/news/detail/09-01-2020-who-statement-regarding-cluster-of-pneumonia-cases-in-wuhan-china. Accessed Febuary 10, 2022.
2. CDC COVID Data Tracker. Centers for Disease Control and Prevention. 2021. Available at: https://covid.cdc.gov/covid-data-tracker/#datatracker-home. Accessed January 4, 2022.
3. Owen WF, Carmona R, Pomeroy C. Failing another national stress test on health disparities. JAMA 2020;323(19):1905.
4. Howell EA, Egorova N, Balbierz A, et al. Black-White differences in severe maternal morbidity and site of care. Am J Obstet Gynecol 2016;214(1):122.e1–7.
5. Artiga S, Hill L, Haldar S. COVID-19 cases and deaths by race/ethnicity: Current data and changes over time. Kaiser Family Foundation; 2022. Available at: https://www.kff.org/racial-equity-and-health-policy/issue-brief/covid-19-cases-and-deaths-by-race-ethnicity-current-data-and-changes-over-time/. [Accessed 1 March 2022].
6. Bunch L. A Tale of Two Crises: Addressing Covid-19 vaccine hesitancy as promoting racial justice. HEC Forum 2021;33(1–2):143–54.
7. Williams DR, Cooper LA. COVID-19 and health equity—a new kind of "herd immunity. JAMA 2020;323(24):2478.
8. Gould E, Wilson V. Black workers face two of the most lethal preexisting conditions for coronavirus—racism and economic inequality. Economic Policy Institute; 2020. Available at: https://files.epi.org/pdf/193246.pdf. [Accessed 4 January 2022].
9. Tyalor B. For Black men, fear that masks will invite racial profiling. New York Times. Available at: https://www.nytimes.com/2020/04/14/us/coronavirus-masks-racism-african-americans.html. Accessed Febuary 10, 2022.
10. Beach MC, Branyon E, Saha S. Diverse patient perspectives on respect in healthcare: a qualitative study. Patient Educ Couns 2017;100(11):2076–80.
11. On behalf of the Harvard Neonatal-Perinatal Fellowship COVID-19 Working Group, Barrero-Castillero A, Beam KS, Bernardini LB, et al. COVID-19: neonatal–perinatal perspectives. J Perinatol 2021;41(5):940–51.
12. Thompson HS, Manning M, Mitchell J, et al. Factors associated with racial/ethnic group–based medical mistrust and perspectives on covid-19 vaccine trial participation and vaccine uptake in the US. JAMA Netw Open 2021;4(5):e2111629.
13. Funk C, Tyyson A. Intent to get a COVID-19 vaccine rise to 60% as confidence in research and development process increases. Pew Research Center; 2020. Available at: https://www.pewresearch.org/science/wp-content/uploads/sites/16/

2020/12/PS_2020.12.03_covid19-vaccine-intent_REPORT.pdf. [Accessed 4 January 2022].

14. Vaccines and related biological products advisory committee meeting December 10, 2020 FDA briefing document Pfizer-BioNTech COVID-19 vaccine. Pfizer and BioNTech. 2020. Available at: https://www.fda.gov/media/144245/download.
15. Center for Disease Control. Health equity considerations and racial and ethnic minority groups. Center for Diease Control; 2022. Available at: https://www.cdc.gov/coronavirus/2019-ncov/community/health-equity/race-ethnicity.html. [Accessed 10 February 2022].
16. US Coronavirus Vaccine Tracker. USA FACTS; January 27th. Available at: https://usafacts.org/visualizations/covid-vaccine-tracker-states/. Accessed June 27, 2022.
17. Ndugga, et al. Latest Data on COVID-19 Vaccinations by race/ethnicity. 2022. Available at: https://www.kff.org/coronavirus-covid-19/issue-brief/latest-data-on-covid-19-vaccinations-by-race-ethnicity/. Accessed January 27, 2022.
18. Khubchandani J, Macias Y. COVID-19 vaccination hesitancy in Hispanics and African-Americans: a review and recommendations for practice. Brain Behav Immun - Health 2021;15:100277.
19. Ellington S, Strid P, Tong VT, et al. Characteristics of women of reproductive age with laboratory-confirmed SARS-CoV-2 Infection by pregnancy status — United States, January 22–June 7, 2020. MMWR Morb Mortal Wkly Rep 2020;69(25):769–75.
20. Mullins E, Hudak ML, Banerjee J, et al. Pregnancy and neonatal outcomes of COVID-19: coreporting of common outcomes from PAN-COVID and AAP-SONPM registries. Ultrasound Obstet Gynecol 2021;57(4):573–81.
21. Adhikari EH, Moreno W, Zofkie AC, et al. Pregnancy outcomes among women with and without severe acute respiratory syndrome coronavirus 2 infection. JAMA Netw Open 2020;3(11):e2029256.
22. MacDorman MF. Race and ethnic disparities in fetal mortality, preterm birth, and infant mortality in the United States: an overview. Semin Perinatol 2011;35(4):200–8.
23. Holness NA, Barfield L, Burns VL, et al. Pregnancy and postpartum challenges during COVID-19 for African-African women. J Natl Black Nurses Assoc 2020;31(2):15–24.
24. Sutton D, D'Alton M, Zhang Y, et al. COVID-19 vaccine acceptance among pregnant, breastfeeding, and nonpregnant reproductive-aged women. Am J Obstet Gynecol MFM 2021;3(5):100403.
25. Leonard SA, Main EK, Scott KA, et al. Racial and ethnic disparities in severe maternal morbidity prevalence and trends. Ann Epidemiol 2019;33:30–6.
26. Colen CG, Ramey DM, Cooksey EC, et al. Racial disparities in health among nonpoor African Americans and Hispanics: The role of acute and chronic discrimination. Soc Sci Med 2018;199:167–80.
27. Green TL, Zapata JY, Brown HW, et al. Rethinking bias to achieve maternal health equity: changing organizations, not just individuals. Obstet Gynecol 2021;137(5):935–40.
28. Reisinger-Kindle K, Qasba N, Cayton C, et al. Evaluation of rapid telehealth implementation for prenatal and postpartum care visits during the COVID-19 pandemic in an academic clinic in Springfield, Massachusetts, United States of America. Health Sci Rep 2021;4(4):e455.
29. Hamel L, Lopes L, Munana C, Artiga S, Brodie M, KFF. Race, health, and COVID 19: The views and experiences of Black Americans., . Key findings from the KFF/

Undefeated survey on race and health. Kaiser Family Foundation; 2020. https://files.kff.org/attachment/Report-Race-Health-and-COVID-19-The-Views-and-Experiences-of-Black-Americans.pdf.
30. Wheeler JM, Misra DP, Giurgescu C. Stress and coping among pregnant Black women during the COVID-19 pandemic. Public Health Nurs 2021;38(4):596–602.
31. Desist C, et al. Risk for stillbirth among women with and without COVID-19 at delivery hospitalization — United States, March 2020–September 2021.; 202AD. Available at: https://www.cdc.gov/mmwr/volumes/70/wr/mm7047e1.htm#:~:text=Pregnant%20women%20are%20at%20increased,1%E2%80%933. Accessed Febuary 10, 2022.
32. Giurgescu C, Wong AC, Rengers B, et al. Loneliness and depressive symptoms among pregnant Black women during the COVID-19 pandemic. West J Nurs Res 2022;44(1):23–30.
33. Bohren MA, Hofmeyr GJ, Sakala C, et al. Continuous support for women during childbirth. Cochrane Database Syst Rev 2017;7:CD003766.
34. Gur RE, White LK, Waller R, et al. The disproportionate burden of the COVID-19 pandemic among pregnant Black women. Psychiatry Res 2020;293:113475.

Educators Countering the Impact of Structural Racism on Health Equity

Kenya V. Beard, EdD, AGACNP-BC, CNE, ANEF, FAAN[a,*],
Wrenetha A. Julion, PhD, MPH, RN, CNL, FAAN[b,c],
Roberta Waite, EdD, PMHCNS, ANEF, FAAN[c]

KEYWORDS

- Structural racism • Health equity • Social justice • Nursing educators
- Race-related discourse

KEY POINTS

- Nursing educators play a pivotal role in the nation's goal of ensuring health equity for all as espoused in the Future of Nursing 2020 to 2030 report.
- Students must be prepared as nurse citizens to understand nursing's core ethical principle of social justice.
- Racism characterizes race as an essential, biological variable, which when converted into clinical practice leads to discriminatory care harshly impacting darker melanated persons.
- Clinical experiences that extend beyond acute care settings and follow individuals where illness impacts them, where they live, work, pray, or learn, should be provided to broaden the ways in which students understand and respond to the impact of structural racism and disease.
- Educators, at a minimum, should be able to facilitate discourse that disrupts the roots of structural racism and advances curriculum in a way that prepares future nurses to mitigate bias and stereotypes.

Health equity endorses that all persons are respected equally, and society must exert intentional efforts to eradicate inequities, historical and present-day injustices, and disrupt health care to enable all persons to thrive. Nursing educators play a pivotal role in the nation's goal of ensuring health equity for all as espoused in the Future of Nursing 2020 to 2030: Charting a Path to Achieve Health Equity.[1] In addition, educators must illuminate a key driver of societal inequities, structural racism, which

This article was not supported by grants.
[a] Chamberlain University, 500 West Monroe Street, Suite 28, Chicago, IL 60661, USA; [b] Rush University, 600 S. Paulina, Suite 1080, Chicago, IL 60612, USA; [c] Georgetown University, 3700 Reservoir Road NW, Washington, DC 20007, USA
* Corresponding author.
E-mail address: kbeard@chamberlain.edu

Nurs Clin N Am 57 (2022) 453–460
https://doi.org/10.1016/j.cnur.2022.04.011
nursing.theclinics.com

augments health disparities.[2] Students must be prepared as nurse citizens to understand nursing's core ethical principle of social justice. However, how do educators prepare future nurses to be social influencers of health and structural competence and serve as leaders and activists that are responsive and act to construct practices, policies, and scholarly activities that advance health equity?

The COVID-19 pandemic has ushered in the raw face of structural racism front and center, in full view of society. Nevertheless, not all faculty discuss structural racism with students.[3] As a core upstream driver, structural racism and its impact on society, including health-related concerns, have negligible appearance, space, or communication in academic nursing. To remain silent now with no meaningful change would really be saying something and that "something" is irreconcilable with nursing's values. It is important to direct our attention to what we fundamentally know, that health disparities arise from racism, which is part of the groundwater of the United States. Nursing educators must be steadfast in acknowledging that racism is a system of inequity, a system of practices, policies, and beliefs designed to afford privilege to white-appearing individuals over racialized Black and brown persons.[4] The whiteness of nursing must concede that racism, whether structural or interpersonal, is our problem because racialized dynamics, in clinical and classroom/didactic spaces, are often reenacted.[5] Nurses may perceive the profession as beneficent; however, it is ever clearer today that nursing is not a stand-alone body invulnerable to racial inequities. More accurately, it is an institution tainted by structural racism. The purpose of this article is to amplify the face of structural racism, to amplify how structural racism impacts health care outcomes, and to provide a meaningful way for educators to unmute race-related discourse in the classroom and counter the impact of structural racism on health equity.

THE FACE OF STRUCTURAL RACISM

Historically, the profession of nursing has impeccably replicated structural mechanisms and accepted and endorsed beliefs of the broader dominant society.[6] Demographically, nurses, including nursing educators, are predominantly white racially. These nurses serve as power agents and gatekeepers, deciding who enters academic programs, what content is taught, what approaches are used for teaching, and what theoretic frameworks are underscored during the academic process. For example, racial essentialism propagates innate racial differences. Racism characterizes race as an essential, biological variable that, when converted into clinical practice, leads to discriminatory care harshly impacting darker melanated persons.

Race, frequently taught as an impartial risk factor for disease, is a facilitator of structural inequities stemming from racist policies. Thus, if nursing students learn about health disparities without context, destructive stereotypes become entrenched with them, believing that some people are naturally unhealthier than others. For example, nursing students find themselves relating race with conditions, such as hypertension and sickle cell anemia, or believing that individuals identified as Blacks feel less pain and have thicker skin, which upholds their implicit understanding of race as a biological trait. Nurse educators should not apply race to make suppositions about biological functions in clinical practice. Rather, educators should use pertinent markers of structural vulnerability (ie, structural racism) and discuss racial disparities in health using structural determinants of health framework and absolutely link race as both a social and a power construct.

IMPACT OF STRUCTURAL RACISM ON HEALTH OUTCOMES

Nursing educators must help students truly understand the impact of structural racism on patient populations, communities, and society at large. Structural racism is so deeply rooted in all aspects of health care and health care education that it significantly diminishes patient outcomes. Therefore, nursing educators, practitioners, and researchers must hold structural racism front and center in all aspects of nursing by prioritizing course and clinical experiences. The elements of curricula that either reinforce, or discredit, structural racism influence how students and future nurses treat their patients and can determine efforts to abolish racism in nursing.[7] Similarly, the focus of research, research questions, methodologies, and the diversity of researchers, can serve to either perpetuate or mitigate structural racism in nursing education and policy.[8,9]

Racism can exert both direct and indirect effects on patient outcomes by influencing the health behaviors of racialized groups.[10] For example, race-related stress can indirectly contribute to smoking, drug use, and overeating, which can fuel racial health disparities. The direct effects of racism can be experienced as psychological and physiologic responses, which occur when individuals attempt to respond to and manage racial stress.[10] For example, John Henryism, a term that describes a style of strong coping behaviors, is attributed to African American strategies to address multiple stressors, including racism. Use of these types of coping behaviors can contribute to poor health outcomes.[11]

Structural racism can be revealed in vulnerable populations through interpersonal violence, institutional discrimination, or socioeconomic disadvantage, which can impact health. Outcomes of structural racism include lifelong accumulated disadvantage, concentrated numbers of racialized individuals living in poor and underserved communities, and the enduring impact of living in a society that views racialized individuals as being less than.[12–15] These outcomes contribute to labeling racialized individuals as high risk for a myriad of health conditions (eg, diabetes, cardiovascular disease, infant mortality and morbidity).[9] Educators should provide the appropriate context when teaching students about these disparate outcomes so that patients are not blamed for their disparate outcomes.

The impact of structural racism on the well-being of racialized individuals has been so profound that 3 major nursing organizations (American Nurses Association, American Academy of Nursing, and American Association of Colleges of Nursing) have come out with position statements on racism.[16] Other major health care organizations, such as the American Medical Association, American Psychological Association, and American Journal of Psychiatry, have issued position statements and/or charges to their constituencies to change research and practice to account for the impact of racism on entrenched health and health care disparities.[17]

There are direct financial costs to individuals, systems, and educational settings associated with structural racism.[17] An important cost that can be attributed to structural racism is the basic need for healthy food and clean water.[13] The financial burden attributed to food insecurity is estimated at $167.5 billion a year, and there is an ever-widening gap between racialized individuals and whites, twice as high for racialized groups.[18] The Flint Water crisis highlights the significant social and health-related costs owing to inattention to health in racialized communities.[13] Mental health care provides another example of the cost-related sequela of structural racism. The cost of mental health care when coupled with the costs of prescription medications fuels disparities. Simultaneously, the societal and structural determinants of mental health contribute to maternal depression, anxiety, alcohol use disorder, and posttraumatic stress disorder. Finally, residential segregation contributes to decreased availability of mental health providers and services in racialized communities.[17]

The costs associated with structural racism prevent African Americans from obtaining equal access to resources, such as wealth, employment, income, education, and health care, resulting in racial disparities in health. Income-related inequities at the individual, household, and societal level perpetuate health disparities, despite government efforts to counter them.[12] For example, the 66% wealth gap between African Americans and whites results from racial inequities in homeownership, income, employment, education, and inheritance.[19] Home ownership is the foundational method for building both net and generational wealth.

The disastrous costs associated with structural racism in nursing education are both individual and collective. At a minimum, the individual cost of racism contributes to psychological distress, early departure, and a racially dominant discipline associated with discriminatory practices and exclusive environments.[20] The collective costs of inadequately preparing all nursing students to fully understand the implications of structural racism contribute to the disproportionate health outcomes.

Other forms of structural racism that contribute to increased cost of lives lost and increased cost of health care include the locations where racialized individuals receive health care. Structural racism has contributed to the dearth of quality and affordable health care. For example, research has revealed that as the numbers of African Americans increase in neighborhoods, the number of hospital closures increase. The remaining hospitals that are left to fill the void become strained and potentially less able to provide quality health care.[19] The US health care system distributes care based on ability to pay. Structural racism in employment, wealth, and income can diminish racialized individuals' ability to receive quality health care.[19]

Structural racism contributes to illness and death among racialized groups because of the impact on multiple health conditions, such as cardiovascular disease, hypertension, diabetes, maternal child health, and the COVID-19 pandemic. Lives lost begin in utero and extend throughout the entire lifespan.[10] For example, in a study by Bishop-Royse and colleagues,[21,22] structural racism, as represented through comparisons between families living in predominantly Black and white communities, revealed that individuals identified as Black had the highest infant mortalities. When socioeconomic status and other social determinants of health were taken into consideration, the disparity remained. Social policies, such as firearm-related mortality, and the criminal justice system also shape health and health outcomes. Educators must help learners understand the detrimental cost to human life that can be attributed to structural racism. Furthermore, educators must be prepared to teach students in ways that promote social justice and to act to counter structural racism in education, research, and practice.

At the other end of the life continuum, the COVID-19 pandemic illustrates the impact of structural racism on older racialized individuals. Past and present experiences with structural racism confer accumulated health disadvantage to older adults through disproportionate exposure and weathering. Age-related changes to the immune system and underlying comorbidities that emerge with age contribute to a higher risk of contracting and spreading the virus when exposed. Physical interactions with health care providers or living in long-term care and assisted living facilities also increase potential exposure. During the pandemic, older adults may also avoid medical care and prescriptions owing to fears of contracting COVID-19, which can undermine existing health conditions.

Weathering, which is defined by Geronimus[23(p411)] as "the effects of sustained cultural oppression upon the body," further explains why racialized individuals are more likely to die or experience serious complications from COVID-19 than whites. Individuals who are weathered are perpetually faced with structural challenges, marginalization, and racial slights from society at-large.[23] Geronimus states that weathering can be positive when used as a mechanism to resist marginalization; yet positive weathering can also erode health. She adds that weathering seeps into the cellular level of individuals when they live and age in a racist society and causes them to age prematurely in response to chronic stress. In addition, the physiologic response to these chronic stressors can also lead to increased consumption of fatty and sugary foods and drug cravings. Garcia[(p4)] describes structural racism as "a pre-existing pathological social condition that drives weathering processes resulting in the greater chronic disease burden among Blacks and Latinxs that elevates their risk of health complications and death." Students who are not aware of these pathologic social conditions will be ill prepared to care for racialized individuals and communities. The authors call for a reframing of what and how pathophysiology is taught to nursing students, how advanced practice nurses are prepared to oversee quality care, and how research questions are developed by student investigators conducting research with racialized communities.

TEACHING TOWARD HEALTH EQUITY

Learning how to advance health equity does not begin or end inside a classroom. However, the extent to which students learn antiracism principles and adopt behaviors that mitigate health care disparities hinges in part on what is taught, where learning occurs, and how race is contextualized. The Future of Nursing 2020 to 2030 report[24(p230)] states that educators "...need to move beyond teaching abstract principles... They also need to create a truly inclusive and safe educational environment and prepare nurses to care for a diverse population... which requires that they understand issues of racism and systems." In the Essentials: Core Competencies for Professional Nursing Education addition, the American Association of Colleges of Nursing[3(p4)] calls for educators to "ensure an understanding of the intersection of bias, structural racism, and social determinants with health care inequities and promote a call to action." The document asserts that to achieve the goals of equity, nursing programs are asked to provide authentic learning opportunities and make "nursing education equitable and inclusive."[3(p6)] To that end, educators must ensure that learners engage in authentic conversations that mitigate race-related stereotypes.[25]

Learning should occur in settings whereby students have an opportunity to not only recognize structural inequities rooted in racism but also denounce and share meaningful ways to mitigate harmful beliefs and practices. Clinical experiences that extend beyond acute care settings and follow individuals where illness impacts them, where they live, work, pray, or learn, should be provided to broaden the ways in which students understand and respond to the impact of structural racism and disease.

Structural racism has created conditions that contribute to health care disparities, and what is or is not taught about race and racism could perpetuate false beliefs that drive how nurses respond to illness. Indeed, negative beliefs about individuals from minoritized groups contribute to inequities[26,27] and patient dissatisfaction. Are students provided opportunities to recognize and mitigate stereotypes? For example, one textbook highlighted that "racial and ethnic minorities have a higher prevalence and greater burden of diabetes compared with whites, and some minority groups also have higher rates of complications."[(p1307)] The text included lack of knowledge as a contributing factor and concluded with "[b]e alert to the risk for diabetes whenever you are interviewing or assessing people who belong to these higher risk racial or ethnic groups."[p1307] Based on the text, should educators fail to contextualize race and racism, nursing students could be primed to believe that race is a biological construct that induces health care disparities.

Unfortunately, there are nursing textbooks that fail to contextualize race. The use of racial classifications, rather than describing how structural racism impacts outcomes, shrouds the truth behind health care disparities and perpetuates race-based stereotypes. Educators, at a minimum, should be able to facilitate discourse that disrupts the roots of structural racism and advances curriculum in a way that mitigates bias and stereotypes. In response to the previously described textbook scenario, faculty could engage in 6 steps to facilitate discourse that denounces race as a biological construct and advances health equity:

1. Recognize the opportunity to contextualize race
2. Restate what is said or written
3. Remove the stigma away from any one individual
4. Provide an opportunity for learners to reflect on potential biases and how decontextualized information threatens health outcomes
5. Recover by discussing how structural racism operates
6. Rebuild by delegitimizing stereotypes and underscoring actions that align with professional values[28]

First, educators should be racially conscious and sensitive to the ways that textbooks and decontextualized outcomes-based discourse perpetuate race-related disparities and recognize the need to contextualize information that addresses race. Second, after identifying race-related assertions, the information should be restated with the intent to emphasize how race is sometimes used as a proxy for structural racism. Third, the learning environment should cultivate an ethos that seeks greater understanding and discourages the pointing of fingers or shaming of individuals or groups. Next, educators should discuss the way the information is provided, albeit unintentional, and provide students with time to reflect on the implications of believing that race is a biological construct. After a moment of reflection, educators could allow students to recover from the pangs of racism by asking students to discuss how ZIP codes, access to education, employment opportunities, and access to high-quality nutrition contribute to disparate outcomes and how structural racism impacts minoritized groups. Last, students have an opportunity to denounce the use of race as a biological determinant of disparities and rebuild narratives by discussing individual actions that align with the nursing value of justice.

SUMMARY

The shattering blows of structural racism continue to undermine efforts to advance health equity. As public awareness of the ways in which racism impacts patient outcomes heightens, so too should the ways in which educators address disparities. Nursing students should be prepared to uphold and advance the principles of health equity. However, discussing structural racism can ignite a paralyzing fear of saying the wrong thing and result in the muting of voices and a failure of educators to contextualize race-related outcomes.[29] Educators have the power to help counter the impact of structural racism on health equity. Although not a panacea, the 6 steps to facilitate race-related discourse could serve as a launching pad for nursing educators to begin conversations that contextualize race, educate students on the ways that structural racism influences health care outcomes, and uphold the right of all people to achieve their highest level of health.

CLINICS CARE POINTS

The six steps to facilitate race-related discourse include the following prompts:

- Recognize the opportunity to contextualize race.
- Restate what is said or written.
- Remove the stigma away from any one individual.
- Reflect on potential biases and how decontextualized information threatens health outcomes.
- Recover by discussing how structural racism operates.
- Rebuild by delegitimizing stereotypes and underscoring actions that align with professional values.

REFERENCES

1. National Academies of Sciences, Engineering, and Medicine. The future of nursing 2020-2030: charting a path to achieve health equity. Washington, DC: The National Academies Press; 2021.
2. Azar K. The evolving role of nurse leadership in the fight for health equity. Nurse Leader 2021;19(6):571–5. https://doi.org/10.1016/j.mnl.2021.08.006.
3. American Association of Colleges of Nursing. The essentials: core competencies for professional nursing education 2021. https://www.aacnnursing.org/Portals/42/AcademicNursing/pdf/Essentials-2021.pdf.
4. Jones CP. Toward the science and practice of anti-racism: Launching a national campaign against racism. Ethn Dis 2018;28(1):231–4. https://doi.org/10.18865/ed.28. S1.231.
5. Moorley C, Darbyshire P, Serrant L, et al. Dismantling structural racism: nursing must not be caught on the wrong side of history. J Adv Nurs 2020;76:2450–3. https://doi-org.ezproxy2.library.drexel.edu/10.1111/jan.14469.
6. Waite R, Nardi D. Nursing colonialism in America: implications for nursing leadership. J Prof Nurs 2017. https://doi.org/10.1016/j.profnurs.2017.12.013.
7. Villarruel AM, Broome ME. Beyond the naming: institutional racism in nursing. Nurs Outlook 2020;68(4):375–6.
8. Beard K, Iruka IU, Laraque-Arena D, et al. Dismantling systemic racism and advancing health equity throughout research. NAM Perspectives. Washington, DC: National Academies of Medicine; 2022.
9. Thurman WA, Johnson KE, Sumpter DF. Words matter: an integrative review of institutionalized racism in nursing literature. Adv Nurs Sci 2019;42(2):89–108.
10. Harrell CJP, Burford TI, Cage BN, et al. Multiple pathways linking racism to health outcomes. Du Bois Rev 2011;8(1):143–57.
11. DeLilly CR, Flaskerud JH. Discrimination and health outcomes. Issues Ment Health Nurs 2012;33(11):801–4.
12. Nickel NC, Lee JB, Chateau J, et al. Income inequality, structural racism, and Canada's low performance in health equity. Healthc Manage Forum 2018; 31(No. 6):245–51. Sage CA: Los Angeles, CA: SAGE Publications.
13. Hammer PJ. The Flint water crisis, the Karegnondi Water Authority and strategic-structural racism. Crit Sociol 2019;45(1):103–19.
14. Yearby R. The impact of structural racism in employment and wages on minority women's health. Hum Rts 2017;43:75.

15. Iheduru-Anderson K, Shingles RR, Akanegbu C. Discourse of race and racism in nursing: an integrative review of literature. Public Health Nurs 2021;38(1):115–30.
16. Knopf A, Budhwani H, Logie CH, et al. A review of nursing position statements on racism following the murder of George Floyd and other Black Americans. J Assoc Nurses AIDS Care 2021;32(4):453–66.
17. Shim RS. Dismantling structural racism in psychiatry: a path to mental health equity. Am J Psychiatry 2021;178(7):592–8.
18. Odoms-Young AM. Examining the impact of structural racism on food insecurity: implications for addressing racial/ethnic disparities. Fam Community Health 2018;41(Suppl 2 FOOD INSECURITY AND OBESITY):S3.
19. Yearby R. The impact of structural racism in employment and wages on minority women's health. Hum. Rts. 2017;43:75.
20. Iheduru-Anderson K, Shingles RR, Akanegbu C. Discourse of race and racism in nursing: An integrative review of literature. Public Health Nursing 2021;38(1): 115–30.
21. Bishop-Royse J, Lange-Maia B, Murray L, et al. Structural racism, socio-economic marginalization, and infant mortality. Public Health 2021;190:55–61.
22. Garcia MA, Homan PA, García C, et al. The color of COVID-19: structural racism and the disproportionate impact of the pandemic on older Black and Latinx adults. Journals Gerontol Ser B 2021;76(3):e75–80.
23. Geronimus AT. Weathering the pandemic: dying old at a young age from pre-existing racist conditions. Wash Lee J Civ Rts Soc Just 2020;27:409.
24. National Academies of Sciences, Engineering, and Medicine. (2021). *The future of nursing 2020-2030: Charting a path to achieve health equity.* Washington, DC: The National Academies Press.
25. Day L, Beard KV. Meaningful inclusion of diverse voices: the case for culturally responsive teaching in nursing education. J Prof Nurs 2019;35(4):277–81.
26. Institute of Medicine. The nations compelling interest: ensuring diversity in the health-care workforce. Available at:http://www.iom.edu/CMS/3740/4888/18287.aspx. Accessed October 12, 2021.
27. Ignatavicius DD, Workman ML. Medical-Surgical nursing: patient-centered collaborative care. 8th ed. Elsevier, Inc; 2016.
28. Mee Mee CL. Insights from Dr. Kenya Beard on health inequities and multicultural nursing education. Teach Learn Nurs 2021;16(3):A1–2.
29. Beard KV, Julion W. Does race still matter in nursing? The narratives of African-American nursing faculty members. Nurs Outlook 2016;64(6):583–96.

Social Support and Loneliness Among Black and Hispanic Senior Women Experiencing Food Insecurity

The Nurse as Primary, Secondary, and Tertiary Intervention

Tracie Walker Kirkland, DNP, ANP-BC, CPNP[a,*],
Jennifer Woo, PhD, CNM/WHNP, FACNM[b]

KEYWORDS

- Vulnerable populations • COVID-19 • Food insecurity • Loneliness
- Perceived social support • Neuman systems model • Nursing intervention • Stress

KEY POINTS

- When compared with White senior women, Black and Hispanic senior women are more likely to have low or moderately low levels of social support, and to experience food insecurity, which may be exacerbated by loneliness.
- Food insecurity has been linked to negative health outcomes, both directly and indirectly as the result of stress.
- Through the lens of The Neuman Systems Model, nurses are in a position to act as sources of primary, secondary, and tertiary prevention to support the wellness of Black and Hispanic senior women who are food insecure.

INTRODUCTION

The impact of social determinants of health (SDOH) on vulnerable populations, especially during the COVID-19 pandemic, is understudied. Additional research in this area is needed. However, while research is being carried out, interventions to improve health outcomes for vulnerable populations can be considered. The aim of this article

[a] Department of Nursing, University of Southern California, Suzanne Dworak-Peck School of Social Work, Texas Women's University, 1150 South Olive Street, Suite T1100, Los Angeles, CA 90015, USA; [b] Texas Woman's University, T. Boone Pickens Institute of Health Sciences, College of Nursing, 5500 Southwestern Medical Avenue, Dallas, TX 75235, USA
* Corresponding author.
E-mail address: tkirklan@usc.edu

Nurs Clin N Am 57 (2022) 461–475
https://doi.org/10.1016/j.cnur.2022.04.012
0029-6465/22/

is to provide a theoretic framework for nurses to identify pathways for nursing interventions to minimizing the influence of food insecurity, perceived social support, and loneliness on stress and client health. The intervention pathways are delineated through the lens of The Neuman Systems Model.[1] The vulnerable population of interest is Black and Hispanic senior women because, when compared with White senior women, Black and Hispanic senior women are more likely to have low or moderately low levels of social support and to experience food insecurity, which may be exacerbated by loneliness.

Background

Poverty

Historically in the United States, poverty rates among Blacks and Hispanics have been higher than poverty rates for Whites.[2,3] Since the onset of the COVID-19 pandemic in February of 2020, overall poverty rates in the US have increased from 15.3% to 16.7%; without federal stimulus payouts afforded by the CARES Act, the increase would have been greater at 18.0%.[4] When compared with Whites (0.08%), Blacks (1.4%) and Hispanics (2.1%) experienced the greatest increases in poverty rates during the pandemic.[4] Considering these inequities, it is no surprise that compared with White (30.7%) women over the age of 65, Black (50.2%) and Hispanic (48.7%) women in that same age group are more likely to live 200% below poverty.[5] Supplemental poverty measure data showed even higher rates and greater disparity, with 41.4% of White women over the age of 65 living 200% below poverty compared with 64.1% of Black women and 67.4% of Hispanic women in the same age group.[5]

Food Insecurity

Because household income is linked to food insecurity[6,7]—defined as food scarcity[8]—it is not surprising that Blacks and Hispanics are more likely to be food insecure when compared with Whites, and that Black and Hispanic women are more likely to be food insecure when compared with men. Specifically, Blacks (11.5%, 7.6%) and Hispanics (10.7%, 4.9%) are more likely to have low and very low food security, respectively, when compared with Whites (4.6%, 3.3%).[9] Women are also more likely to have low (19.1%) or very low (9.6%) food security when compared with men (9.5%, 5.9%, respectively).[9]

Similar conditions exist for Black women. In 2017, 79.4% of non-Hispanic White women but only 9.0% of non-Hispanic Black women were food secure.[10] Additionally, non-Hispanic Black women were more likely to be food insecure (22.8%) than to be food secure (9.0%).[10] Furthermore, Black (15.1%) and Hispanic (14.8%) seniors age 60 and older are more likely to be food insecure when compared with White (6.2%) seniors in the same age group.[11]

Loneliness and Social Support

For women, food insecurity has been linked with social support[10] and the social capital those supports provide.[12] Most of the women who are food insecure have low (59.1%) or moderate (31.0%) levels of social support.[10] Marital status,[13] participation in a government assistance program,[13,14] household income (ie, poverty),[6] education,[15] employment,[16] and loneliness[13,14] are additional factors of food insecurity. During the COVID-19 pandemic, seniors have reported experiencing increased loneliness.[17,18]

RATIONALE

Loneliness has been linked to negative health outcomes, including depression for those who developed closer relationships within their social networks during the pandemic.[18] Food insecurity has been linked generally to overall poorer self-reported health[7,19] as well as to prediabetes,[6,20–22] diabetes,[7,21,23] high blood pressure, congestive heart failure, heart attack, asthma,[7] obesity,[24] and nonalcoholic fatty liver disease.[25]

Comorbidities may negatively mediate the influence of food insecurity on health outcomes.[26] Comorbidities include cardiovascular disease,[27,28] cancer,[27,29] chronic fatigue syndrome,[30] musculoskeletal injury,[31] and depression,[27,32] and health-related behaviors include smoking, substance abuse, and poor[27] and disturbed eating habits.[33]

Enrollment in a nutrition assistance program may mediate the influence of low food security on overall physical health outcomes.[19,34] Additionally, social support[35]—potentially in the form of nursing prevention interventions[35]—can reduce the influence of comorbidities and health-related behaviors[27] and thus act as a barrier against the adverse effects of stress on patient health.[35]

The specific focus on Black and Hispanic populations is warranted not only because of the greater potential for those populations to be socioeconomically challenged[2,3] and food insecure[9,11] but also because Blacks and Hispanics have been found to have higher incidence of stress when compared with Whites.[27] Sources of stress disparity include (a) greater exposure to incidents of discrimination[36] and violence, (b) greater exposure to barriers to occupational advancement,[37] and (c) the cultivation of resources useful for overcoming these sources of stress[38] have been exacerbated with the COVID 19 pandemic.

THE CLIENT SYSTEM

The Neuman systems model is based on the concept of the client system, which can be considered a single client, a group, or multiple groups, and is focused on how those systems interact with their environments[39] in response "to actual or potential environmental stressors, and the use of primary, secondary, and tertiary nursing prevention interventions for retention, attainment, and maintenance of optimal client system wellness."[35(p67)] Types of environmental stressors vary[39] and can be "intrapersonal, interpersonal, and extrapersonal" and characteristically "physiologic, psychological, sociocultural, developmental, and spiritual."[35(p67)] Examples of stressors include "loss, pain, sensory deprivation, [and] cultural change".[39(p20)]

Levels of Energy

In the client system model, available energy for resisting stressors exists in 3different capacities and in addition to basic bodily functions such as genetic structure, organ strength and weakness, and body temperature regulation.[39] Those levels of energy within client systems are referred to as lines of resistance, normal lines of defense, and flexible lines of defense. In all cases, a client's levels of energy are supported by coping mechanisms, cultural and spiritual belief systems, and lifestyle factors.

A client's normal line of defense refers to the client's usual state of wellness and is developed and shaped over time through client behaviors.[39] The client's usual state of wellness, defined as the stable condition of the client system, serves as a baseline for assessing deviances from that condition.

When a client's normal line of defense is disrupted, the client's lines of resistance are activated whereby the client's internal and external resources (both known and unknown) engage to protect the client against the identified encroaching stressor.[39] The client's lines of resistance include major biological protection systems such as the immune system's activation of white blood cells in response to injury or infection. Ideally, the client's lines of resistance will be sufficient enough to return the client system to a stable condition. The alternative is the depletion of system energy and client death.

A client's flexible line of defense is their primary protective element against environmental stressors that disrupt the client's normal line of defense (ie, stable health).[39] The client's flexible line of defense is dynamic and can fluctuate rapidly. A simplified graphic of the Neuman systems model is presented in **Fig. 1**.

Client Perceptions of Health

In addition to client system reactions to stressors, the ways in which clients perceive their health[35] and the way they cope with stressors[39] influences the strength of their lines of defense and resistance. Essentially, stress is a neutral concept that only gains the capacity for positive or negative influences on health outcomes to the degree that the client perceives the stressor will have positive or negative outcomes and to the extent that the client perceives they are capable of coping with the stressor.[35,39] The mere exposure to a pandemic is a stressor for the client. Couple this with systemic racism and lack of resources, this potentiates stress affecting lines of defense. The concepts of client perceptions and coping are rooted in Lazarus and Folkman's theory of stress and coping.

Stress and Coping

Unlike traditional, and dichotomous, perspectives of stress that characterize stress as either a stimulus or response, Lazarus and Folkman[35] considered stress a factor related to the characteristics of both the person and the environment for which the person functions. This relationship between stress and the characteristics of both the person and the environment for which the person functions is similar to the way

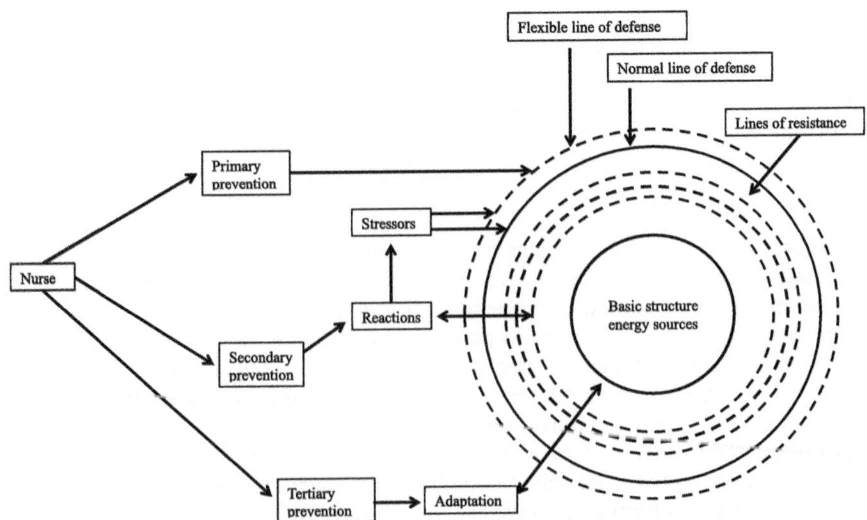

Fig. 1. Simplified interpretation of the Neuman systems model. (*Note. Adapted from* The Neuman Systems Model, by B. Neuman and J. Fawcett, 2011 (5th ed.), p. 13, Pearson.)

illness cannot be considered solely a function of external influences but a combination of those influences and a person's behavior and susceptibility to illness. Central and critical components to managing stress are appraisal and coping, whereas the degree to which a person perceives a situation to be stressful (appraisals) and that that person can successfully cope with that stressor is due, in part, to that person's perceived level of social support. Subsequently, the person's perceived the stressfulness of a situation and their capacity to cope with the stressful situation influences the person's ability to adapt to the stressful situation. Finally, a person's ability to adapt to a stressful situation mediates the influence of stress on a person's health outcomes. In this way, social support encourages a relationship perspective that can protect people from the negative health outcomes associated with stress.[40] Additionally, from this perspective, people with greater levels of perceived social support will be less likely to experience stress-related health problems because they will be less likely to judge their situations as stressful.

Primary, Secondary, and Tertiary Roles of the Nurse

Because the Neuman systems model can be applied to a variety of populations and conditions, it is uniquely adaptable to a range of health care concerns in nursing and can be used to delineate the primary, secondary, and tertiary roles of the nurse within the client system.[39] Primary preventions are those that occur before a client encounters and reacts to a stressor. Nursing actions that can function as primary preventions are associated with general nursing knowledge used to identify and assess potential client stressors and implement interventions to mitigate or alleviate those stressors. Additionally, primary preventions may be focused on increasing a client's flexible lines of defense.

Secondary preventions are those that occur after a client encounters and reacts to a stressor.[39] Nursing actions that can function as secondary preventions are associated with symptomology related to client reactions to stressors. Actions in this category of prevention include prioritizing interventions and implementing interventions focused on reducing the negative effects of clients' reactions to stressors. Interventions of this nature might include early screening and detection, and treatment of symptoms.

Tertiary preventions are those that occur after a client has reacted to a stressor and received treatment.[39] Nursing actions that can function as tertiary preventions are those that help clients adjust and adapt to changing health conditions and move clients closer to system stability. Interventions of this nature might include education meant to prevent future susceptibility to a particular stressor.

CONCEPTUAL APPLICATION OF THE NEUMAN SYSTEM MODEL

In this article, the Neuman systems model is used to consider food insecurity as a source of stress for the client system, in this case, the Black or Hispanic female senior patient who is food insecure. Perceived social support and loneliness are considered factors of food insecurity. The nurse is conceptualized as a source of primary, secondary, and tertiary interventions. A graphic representation of the relationships among the theoretic concepts presented to this point and the associated covariates and mediating factors is presented in **Fig. 2**.

The holistic perspective of the Neuman systems model makes it not only "timeless [but] expansive in being adaptable to all client care situations."[41(p112)] Because the client system is dynamic, nurses may effectually help transform those systems to promote better health outcomes for clients. Using the Neuman systems model to examine the relationships between perceived social support, loneliness, and food insecurity

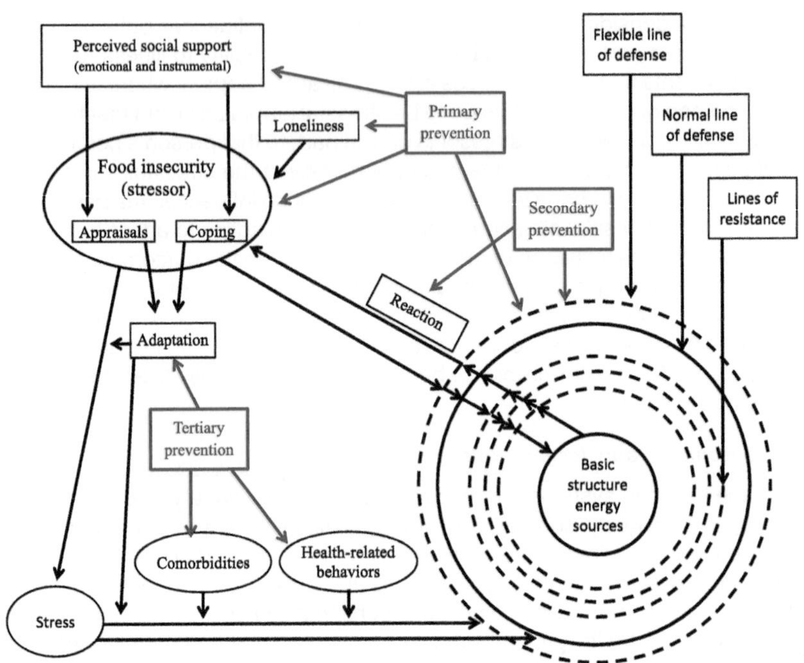

Fig. 2. Application of the Neuman systems model: Food insecurity as a stressor on the client system.

provides an effective means not only for considering the patient as a complex system but for understanding how the environment influences that system and the varied ways in which nurses can serve as sources of support for patient wellness.

As initiators of preventions in the food insecure client senior minority model, nurses may direct clients to sources of emotional and instrumental support and companionship. They also may function to help clients improve their perceptions about their experiences with food insecurity and to better adapt to outcomes of the food insecurity they are experiencing, including stress. Additionally, nurses may help promote client engagement in positive health-related behaviors while also addresses comorbidities that may be having additional negative influences on the client system. In these ways, nurses have the capacity to contribute to improved client wellness, in this case, specifically Black and Hispanic senior women who are food insecure.

APPLICATION IN PRACTICE

A list of suggested primary, secondary, and tertiary preventions and their conceptualized applications in practice as they relate to perceived social support, loneliness, and food insecurity is presented in **Table 1**. These suggestions are not all inclusive, and nurses are encouraged to generate other potential means of prevention. Nurses conduct health assessments and obtain data related to the psycho-social-cultural being which allows one to examine potential risks for allostatic load and burden of diseases. Early detection is key and providing a toolkit for vulnerable populations in particular to have during unplanned circumstances such as pandemics and or natural disasters may be key elements in attaining good health outcomes.

Table 1
The nurse as source of primary, secondary, and tertiary prevention

Model Component	Application in Practice
Primary prevention	
Identify and assess potential client stressors	• Identify food insecurity as a potential stressor to the client system • Assess the degree to which food insecurity has the potential to negatively affect the client system • Identify social support and loneliness as potential influences on client's perceived severity of food insecurity • Assess the degree to which social support and loneliness are potential influences on client's perceived severity of food insecurity
Primary prevention	
Implement interventions to mitigate or alleviate those stressors	• Generation of food assistance program database and educational materials for clients • Generation of emotional and instrumental support program database and educational materials for clients • Generation of companionship program database and educational materials for clients
Increase client's line of flexible defense	• Through primary preventions focused on decreasing experiences of food insecurity • Through primary preventions focused on decreasing experiences of low emotional and instrumental support • Through primary preventions focused on decreasing experiences of loneliness • Client perception that the nurse is a source of social support
Secondary prevention	
Prioritize interventions and implement interventions focused on reducing the negative effects of clients' reactions to stressors	• Formal screening for food insecurity • Informal screening for lack of social support and signs of loneliness • Referral to support services: food, emotional support, instrumental support, and companionship programs • Encourage client use of support services • Encourage support seeking behavior • Encourage engagement in positive health-related behaviors • Support behaviors to minimize or eliminate comorbidities
Tertiary prevention	
• Promote client adjustment and adaptation to changing health conditions	Encourage positive thought patterns

(*continued on next page*)

Table 1
(*continued*)

Model Component	Application in Practice
• Nurture client journey to system stability ∘ Looking at feedback on secondary prevention ∘ Reeducation to prevent the recurrence of stressors	• Analyze the effectiveness of screening for food insecurity, social support, and loneliness • If interventions are effective, remind nurse colleagues about available client supports to prevent future occurrences of stressors • Analyze value of referrals for food programs, emotional support programs, instrumental support programs, and companionship programs • If interventions are effective, remind clients about the available support programs • Analyze the effectiveness of encouraging client use of support services, support seeking behavior, and engagement in positive health-related behaviors
Tertiary prevention	
• Nurture client journey to system stability ∘ Looking at the feedback on secondary prevention ∘ Reeducation to prevent recurrence of stressors	• If interventions are effective, remind nurse colleagues about the value of encouraging these client behaviors • Analyze the effectiveness of supporting client behaviors to minimize or eliminate comorbidities • If interventions are effective, remind nurse colleagues of the value of encouraging client behaviors to minimize or eliminate comorbidities
Support maintenance of healthy client system	Return to primary prevention processes

RECOMMENDATIONS

Some of the preventions suggested in **Table 1**, in particular those that require identification and assessment, necessitate the observation and/or measure of social support, loneliness, and food insecurity. Nurses are urged to consider the various definitions of these terms as they plan potential interventions. A list is provided in **Table 2**, although this list is not inclusive. Because of the conceptual complexity of social support and food insecurity, those terms are discussed in more detail.

Social Support

Over the last 4 decades, researchers and theorists have proposed various definitions of social support in response to their explorations of its connection to psychological and physical manifestations of health.[45,50] Lack of agreement on the definition is due to its multidimensionality in the way it operates,[43] whereas support can be (a) both given and received, (b) considered from the perspectives of both availability and use, and (c) considered from the perspective of the origin of the support.[51] However, social support also can be informal or formal[52] and emotional or instrumental.[42] Social support also can be considered with respect to clinical utility and health outcomes,[52] whereas social support can be a direct influence on health outcomes or a

Table 2
Definition of terms

Variable	Definition
Social support	
NIH Toobox,[42(p28)]	Social relationships that are "available to provide aid in times of need or when problems arise"
Shumaker & Brownell[43(p11)]	"An exchange of resources between at least 2 individuals perceived by the provider or the recipient to be intended to enhance the well-being of the recipient"
Cohen[44(p676)]	"A social network's provision of psychological and material resources intended to benefit an individual's ability to cope with stress" (p. 676)
Feeney & Collins[45(p1)]	"Deep and meaningful close relationships"
Loneliness	
NIH Toolbox,[42(p28)]	"Perceptions that one is alone, lonely or socially isolated from others"
De Jong Gierveld & Van Tilburg[46]	The feeling of missing an intimate relationship (emotional loneliness) or missing a wider social network (social loneliness)
Food Insecurity	
Operational	
Johnson et al.[47(p1257)]	Food insecurity measured by the 4 domains of the Four Domain Food Insecurity Scale: "shortage of food (quantitative), unsuitability of food and diet (qualitative), preoccupation or uncertainty in access to enough food (psychological), and alienation or lack of control over their food situation (social)"
Conceptual	
Anderson[48(1560)]	"Food insecurity exists whenever the availability of nutritionally adequate and safe foods or the ability to acquire acceptable foods in socially acceptable ways is limited or uncertain"
Murillo et al.[8(p428)]	"Lack of access or availability to healthy foods due to scarce resources or money"
Nagarajan et al.[49]	Lack of availability of healthy foods
Wright et al.[22(p130)]	"Limited access to a sufficient quantity of affordable, nutritious food"

buffering agent such that social support lessens the negative outcomes associated with stressful events.[53]

Food Insecurity

The United States Department of Agriculture (USDA) typically refers to food security, which they define as "access by all people at all times to enough food for an active, healthy life"[9(p2)] Murillo and colleagues[8] referred to that USDA definition for food security when they defined its opposite, food insecurity. As shown in **Table 2**, Wright and colleagues[22] and Nagarajan and colleagues[49] defined food insecurity using similar language. However, unlike Murillo and colleagues who included reasons for the lack of access to or availability of healthy foods in their definition of food insecurity, neither

Wright nor Nagarajan and colleagues do so. The USDA also does not reference reasons for having access to enough food in its definition of food security. The most comprehensive definition of food insecurity includes quantitative, qualitative, psychological, and social factors associated with food insecurity.[47] Because it is broad in scope, that definition is suggested for use in future research.

SUMMARY

A disciplinary focus in the nursing field is social justice; as nurses, we are morally obligated to act in ways that promote immediate social change in the form of improved patient care and outcomes.[54] Nurses are in an ideal position to examine SDOH and to implement strategies to rectify health inequities among vulnerable groups such as the aging population. Additionally, nurse educators are well-situated to raise awareness of the importance of nurses to act in this capacity. Such efforts are encouraged and could help the United States move closer to the 2030 goal of eradicating food insecurity championed by the Food and Agriculture Organization of the United Nations and colleagues[55] and reducing the incidence of health inequities among Black and Hispanic senior women.

In addition to improving patient outcomes, reduction of cost negative health-related outcomes of food insecurity could be reduced. According to Berkowitz and colleagues,[56] median annual state- and county-level health care costs are $687,041,000 and $4,433,000, respectively. For food insecure adults, additional health care costs amount to $1834 annually. At the national level, those numbers are even more astounding at $77.5 billion and $1,863, respectively.[57] Saved monies could be reallocated for additional interventions to further reduce the incidence of health inequities among Black and Hispanic senior women.

The timing of this article correlates with the updated recommendations put forth in *The Essentials: Core Competencies for Professional Nursing Education* which include SDOH as one of the 8 featured concepts for professional nursing education programs.[58] The 8 concepts are intertwined among 10 domains of competence; together, they represent what the American Association of Colleges of Nursing describes as a new model for nursing education that is competency based, structured for application across levels of education, and adaptable to accommodate a future change in the field of nursing.

The inclusion of SDOH as an essential concept of learning for nurses underscores the important role nurses can serve in addressing SDOH and health inequities that contribute to inequity in health outcomes. Through health and needs assessments, health promotion, patient education, and improved access to care, nurses may have a direct impact on the health care of community members from vulnerable populations.[58] In this article, we argued that these very actions be taken by nurses acting as primary, secondary, and tertiary interventions to improve health outcomes for Black and Hispanic senior women experiencing food insecurity.

CLINICS CARE POINTS

Screening for SDOH during the patient intake process can be expedited using

- The Hunger Vital Sign screening tool (2 items),[59]
- The Three-Item Loneliness Scale,[60] and
- The Social Support Questionnaire (SSQ3; three-item short form).[61]

Referral to food support programs is associated with decreased

- Loneliness,[62]
- Medication nonadherence,[63]
- Admissions to nursing homes,[64] and
- Overall health care costs.[65]

DISCLOSURE

The authors have nothing to disclose.

REFERENCES

1. Neuman B. The Neuman systems model in research and practice. Nurs Sci Q 1996;9(2):67–70. https://doi.org/10.1177/089431849600900207.
2. Chaudry A, Wimer C, Macartney S, et al. Poverty in the United States: 50-year trends and safety net impacts. Office of human services policy, office of the assistant secretary for planning and evaluation. U.S. Department of Health and Human Services; 2016. https://aspe.hhs.gov/system/files/pdf/154286/50YearTrends.pdf.
3. Semega J, Kollar M, Shrider EA, et al. *Income and Poverty in the United States: 2019* (report No. P60-270). U. S. Department of Commerce, U. S. Census Bureau; 2020. https://www.census.gov/content/dam/Census/library/publications/2020/demo/p60-270.pdf.
4. Parolin Z, Curran M, Matsudaira J, et al. Monthly poverty rates in the United States during the COVID-19 pandemic. Center on Poverty and Social Policy; 2020. https://www.povertycenter.columbia.edu/s/COVID-Projecting-Poverty-Monthly-CPSP-2020.pdf.
5. Cubanski J, Koma W, Damico A, et al. H*ow many seniors Live in poverty?* Kaiser Family Foundation; 2020. http://files.kff.org/attachment/Issue-Brief-How-Many-Seniors-Live-in-Poverty.
6. Lee AM, Scharf RJ, Filipp SL, et al. Food insecurity is associated with prediabetes risk among U.S. adolescents, NHANES 2003–2014. Metab Syndr Relat Disord 2019;17(7):347–54. https://doi.org/10.1089/met .2019.0006.
7. Ziliak JP, Gundersen C. The health consequences of senior hunger in the United States: evidence from the 1999-2014 NHANES. Feeding America and the National Foundation to End Senior Hunger; 2017. https://www.feedingamerica.org/sites/default/files/research/senior-hunger-research/senior-health-consequences-2014.pdf.
8. Murillo R, Reesor LM, Scott CW, et al. Food insecurity and pre-diabetes in adults: race/ethnic and sex differences. Am J Health Behav 2017;41(4):428–36. https://doi.org/10.5993/AJHB.41.4.7.
9. Coleman-Jensen A, Rabbitt MP, Gregory CA, et al. *Household food Security in the United States in 2019* (economic research report No. 275). United States Department of Agriculture; 2020. https://www.ers.usda.gov/webdocs/publications/99282/err-275.pdf?v=3572.4.
10. Ashe KM, Lapane KL. Food insecurity and obesity: exploring the role of social support. J Women's Health 2018;27(5):651–8. https://doi.org/10.1089/jwh.2017.6454.
11. Ziliak JP, Gundersen C. The state of senior hunger in America in 2018. Feeding America; 2020. Available at: https://www .feedingamerica.org/sites/default/files/2020-05/2020-The%20State%20of%20Senior%20 Hunger%20in%202018.pdf.

12. Leedy AM, Whittle HJ, Shieh J, et al. Exploring the role of social capital in managing food insecurity among older women in the United States. Soc Sci Med 2020;265:1–8. https://doi.org/10.1016/j .socscimed.2020.113492.
13. Burris M, Kihlstrom L, Serrano Arce K, et al. Food insecurity, loneliness, and social support among older adults. J Hunger Environ Nutr 2021;16(1):29–44. https://doi.org/10.1080/19320248.2019.1595253.
14. Hunt BR, Benjamins MR, Khan S, et al. Predictors of food insecurity in selected Chicago community areas. J Nutr Educ Behav 2018;51(3):287–99. https://doi.org/10.1016/j.jneb.2018.08.005.
15. Tarasuk V, Fafard St-Germain A-A, Mitchell A. Geographic and sociodemographic predictors of household food insecurity in Canada, 2011–12. BMC Public Health 2019;19(1):1–12. https://doi.org/10.1186/s12889-018-6344-2.
16. Reeves A, Loopstra R, Tarasuk V. Wage-setting policies, employment, and food insecurity: a multilevel analysis of 492 078 people in 139 countries. Am J Public Health 2021;111(4):718–25. https://doi.org/10.2105/AJPH.2020.306096.
17. Kotwal A, Holt-Lunstad J, Newmark RL, et al. Social isolation and loneliness among San Francisco Bay Area older adults during the COVID-19 shelter-in-place orders. J Am Geriatr Soc 2020;69(1):20–9. https://doi.org/10.1111/jgs.16865.
18. Krendl AC, Perry BL. The impact of sheltering in place during the COVID-19 pandemic on older adults' social and mental well-being. J Gerontol B Psychol Sci 2020;76(2):e53–8. https://doi.org/10.1093/geronb/gbaa110.
19. Pak T-Y, Kim G. Food stamps, food insecurity, and health outcomes among elderly Americans. Prev Med 2020;130:1–7. https://doi.org/10.1016/j.ypmed.2019.105871.
20. Lee AM, Scharf RJ, DeBoer MD. Food insecurity is associated with prediabetes and dietary differences in U. S. adults aged 20-39. Prev Med 2018;116:180–5. https://doi.org/10.1016/j.ypmed.2018.09.012.
21. Walker RJ, Grusnik J, Garacci E, et al. Trends in food insecurity in the USA for individuals with prediabetes, undiagnosed diabetes, and diagnosed diabetes. J Gen Intern Med 2018;34(1):33–5. https://doi.org/10.1007/s11606-018-4651-z.
22. Wright L, Stallings-Smith S, Arikawa AY. Associations between food insecurity and prediabetes in a representative sample of U.S. adults (NHANES 2005-2014). Diabetes Res Clin Pract 2019;148:130–6. https://doi.org/10.1016/j.diabres.2018 .11.017.
23. Tarr K, Weber M, Holben D. Food insecurity and Type 2 diabetes risk of adults with school children [Abstract]. J Acad Nutr Diet 2018;118(9, suppl. 1):A-74. https://doi.org/10.1016/j.jand.2018.06.048.
24. Kaiser ML, Cafer A. Understanding high incidence of severe obesity and very low food security in food pantry clients: Implications for social work. Soc Work Public Health 2018;33(2):125–39. https://doi.org/10.1080/19371918.2017 .1415181.
25. Golovaty I, Tien PC, Price CJ, et al. Food insecurity may be an independent risk factor associated with nonalcoholic fatty liver disease among low-income adults in the United States. J Nutr 2019;150(1):91–8. https://doi.org/10.1093/jn/nxz212.
26. Palakshappa D, Speiser JL, Rosenthal GE, et al. Food insecurity is associated with an increased prevalence of comorbid medical conditions in obese adults: NHANES 2007–2014. J Gen Intern Med 2019;34:1486–93. https://doi .org/10.1007/s11606-019-05081-9.
27. American Psychological Association. Stress and health disparities. Contexts, mechanisms, and interventions among racial/ethnic minority and socioeconomic

status populations. American Psychological Association; 2021. https://www.apa.org/pi/health-disparities/resources/stress-report.pdf.
28. Schnall PL, Dobson M, Landsbergis P. Globalization, work, and cardiovascular disease. Int J Health Serv 2016;46(4):656–92.
29. Johansen C, Sørensen IK, Høeg BL, et al. Stress and cancer. In: Cooper CL, Quick JC, editors. The Handbook of Stress and health. A Guide to Research and practice. Blackwell; 2017. p. 125–34.
30. Grinde B. Stress and chronic fatigue syndrome. In: Cooper CL, Quick JC, editors. The Handbook of Stress and health. A Guide to Research and practice. Blackwell; 2017. p. 135–46.
31. Hartzell MM, Dodd CDT, Gatchel RJ. Stress and musculoskeletal injury. In: Cooper CL, Quick JC, editors. The handbook of stress and health. A guide to research and practice. Blackwell; 2017. p. 201–22.
32. Lerner D, Adler DA, Rogers WH, et al. The double burden of work stress and depression: a workplace intervention. In: Cooper CL, Quick JC, editors. The handbook of stress and health. A guide to research and practice. Blackwell; 2017. p. 147–67.
33. Bennett DA. Stress and eating disturb behavior. In: Cooper CL, Quick JC, editors. The handbook of stress and health. A guide to research and practice. Blackwell; 2017. p. 186–209.
34. McLain AC, Xiao RS, Gao X, et al. Food insecurity and odds of high allostatic load in Puerto Rican adults: the role of participation in the Supplemental Nutrition Assistance Program during 5 years of follow-up. Psychosom Med 2018;80(8): 733–41. https://doi.org/10.1097/PSY.00000000000 00628.
35. Lazarus RS, Folkman S. Stress, coping, and appraisal. Springer; 1984.
36. Sternthal MJ, Slopen N, Williams DR. Racial disparities in health. Du Bois Rev 2011;8:95–113. https://doi.org/10.1017/S1742 058X11000087.
37. Browning CR, Calder CA, Ford JL, et al. Understanding racial differences in exposure to violent areas: integrating survey, smartphone, and administrative data resources. Ann Am Acad Pol Soc Sci 2017;669(1):41–62. https://doi.org/10.1177/0002716216678167.
38. Lewis TT, Cogburn CD, Williams DR. Self-reported experiences of discrimination and health: Scientific advances, ongoing controversies, and emerging issues. Annu Rev Clin Psychol 2015;11:407–40. https://doi.org/10.1146/annurev-linpsy-032814-112728.
39. Neuman B, Fawcett J. The neuman systems model. 5th ed. Pearson; 2011.
40. Lackey B, Cohen S. Social support theory and selecting measures of social support. In: Cohen S, Gordon LU, Gottlieb BH, editors. Social support measurement and interventions: a guide for health and social scientits. 2000. p. 29–52. Oxford.
41. Newman B, Reed KS. A Neuman systems model perspective on nursing in 2050. Nurs Sci Qt 2007;20(2):111–3. https://doi.org/10.1177/0894318407299847.
42. NIH Toolbox. NIH Toolbox. Scoring and Interpretation Guide for the iPad. 2016. Available at: https://nihtoolbox.my.salesforce.com/sfc/p/2E00 0001H4ee/a/2E0000004yR3/Ckb_AKw1oFUC56tgf6tdxcGDYaYbu8rsmBSFOX2Ec4g. Accessed January 30, 2021.
43. Shumaker SA, Brownell A. Toward a theory of social support: closing conceptual gaps. J Soc Issues 1984;40(4):11–36. https://doi.org/10.1111/j.1540-4560.1984.tb 01105.x.
44. Cohen S. Social relationships and health. Am Psychol 2004;59(8):676–84. https://doi.org/10.1037/0003-066X.59.8.676.

45. Feeney BC, Collins NL. New look at social support: a theoretical perspective on thriving through relationships. Pers Soc Psychol Rev 2015;19(2):113–47. https://doi.org/10.1177/1088868314544222.
46. de Jong Gierveld J, van Tilburg T. The De Jong Gierveld short scales for emotional and social loneliness: tested on data from 7 countries in the UN generations and gender surveys. Eur J Ageing 2010;7(2):121–30. https://doi.org/10.1007/s10433-010-0144-6.
47. Johnson CM, Ammerman AS, Adair LS, et al. The four domain food insecurity scale (4D-FIS): Development and evaluation of a complementary food insecurity measure. Transl Behav Med 2020;10(6):1255–65. https://doi.org/10.1093/tbm/ibaa125.
48. Anderson SA. Core indicators of nutritional state for difficult-to-sample populations. J Nutr 1990;120(suppl. 11):1555–600. https://doi.org/10.1093/jn/120.suppl_11.1555.
49. Nagarajan S, Khokhar A, Sweetnam Holmes D, et al. Family consumer behaviors, adolescent prediabetes and diabetes in the National Health and Nutrition Examination Survey (2007-2010). J Am Coll Nutr 2017;36(7):520–7. https://doi.org/10.1080/07315724.2017.1327828.
50. Zimet GD, Dahlem NW, Zimet SG, et al. The multidimensional scale of perceived social support. J Pers Assess 1988;52(1):30–41. https://doi .org/10.1207/s15327752jpa5201_2.
51. Tardy CH. Social support measurment. Am J Community Psychol 1985;13(2):187–202. https://doi.org/10.1007/BF00905728.
52. Streeter CL, Franklin C. Defining and measuring social support: Guidelines for social work practitioners. Res Soc Work Pract 1992;2(1):81–98. https://doi .org/10.1177/104973159200200107.
53. Cohen S, Wills TA. Stress, social support, and the buffering hypothesis. Psychol Bull 1985;98(2):310–57. https://doi.org/10.1037/0033-2909.98.2.310.
54. Dillard-Wright J, Shields-Hass V. Nursing with people. Reimagining future for nursing. Adv Nurs Sci 2021. https://doi.org/10.1097/ANS.0000000000000361. Advance online publication:.
55. Food and Agriculture Organization of the United Nations, International Fund for Agricultural Development, UNICEF, World Food Programme, & World Health Organization. The state of food security and nutrition in the world. Transforming food systems for affordable healthy diets. food and agriculture organization of the United Nations, international fund for agricultural development, UNICEF. World Food Programme, & World Health Organization; 2020. https://doi.org/10.4060/ca9692en.
56. Berkowitz SA, Basu S, Gundersen C, et al. State-level and county- level estimates of health care costs associated with food insecurity. Prev Chronic Dis 2019;16. https://doi.org/10.5888/pcd16.180549.
57. Berkowitz SA, Basu S, Meigs JB, et al. Food insecurity and health care expenditures in the United States, 2011–2013. Health Ser Res 2018;53(3):1600–20. https://doi.org/10.1111/1475-6773.12730.
58. American Association of Colleges of Nursing. The essentials: Core competencies for professional nursing education. American Association of Colleges of Nursing; 2021. Available at: https://www.aacnnursing.org/Portals/42/AcademicNursing/pdf/Essentials-2021.pdf. Accessed December 14, 2021.
59. Gundersen C, Engelhard EE, Crumbaugh AS, et al. Brief assessment of food insecurity accurately identifies high-risk US adults. Public Health Nutr 2017;20(8):1367–71. https://doi.org/10.1017/S1368980017000180.

60. Hughes ME, Waite L, Hawkley LC, et al. A short scale for measuring loneliness in large surveys: Results from two population-based studies. Res Aging 2004;26(6): 655–72. https://doi.org/10.1177/0164027504268574.
61. Sarason IG, Sarason BR, Shearin EN, et al. A brief measure of social support: Practical and theoretical implications. J Soc Pers Relat 1987;4:497–510. https://doi.org/10.1177/0265407587044007.
62. Thomas KS, Akobundu U, Dosa D. Gerontol B Psychol Sci Soc Sci 2016;71(6): 1049–58. https://doi.org/10.1093/geronb/gbv111.
63. Srinivasan M, Pooler JA. Cost-related medication nonadherence for older adults participating in SNAP, 2013-2015. Am J Public Health 2018;108(2):224–30. https://doi.org/10.2105/AJPH.2017.304176.
64. Szanton SL, Samuel LJ, Cahill R, et al. Food assistance is associated with decreased nursing home admissions for Maryland's dually eligible older adults. BMC Geriatr 2017;17(1):162. https://doi.org/10.1186/s12877-017-0553-x.
65. Berkowitz SA, Seligman HK, Rigdon J, et al. Supplemental nutrition assistance program (SNAP) participation and health care expenditures among low-income adults. JAMA Intern Med 2017;177(11):1642–9. https://doi.org/10.1001/jamainternmed.2017.4841.

Opioid Overdose Harm Prevention

The Role of the Nurse in Patient Education

Selena Gilles, DNP, ANP-BC, CNEcl, FNYAM

KEYWORDS

- Overdose prevention • Harm reduction • Pain management • Naloxone
- Opioid overdose

KEY POINTS

- Opioid overdose continues to take thousands of lives each year in the United States. To reverse this epidemic, we need to not only improve the way we treat pain, but also implement effective evidence-based measures that prevent misuse, addiction, and overdose.
- Nurses, as members of the health care team, are uniquely positioned as direct patient care providers, patient educators, patient advocates, and leaders to play a critical role in these efforts.
- Nurses should become familiar with the many local and federal initiatives to combat opioid misuse and overdose including conducting surveillance and research, better addiction, treatment and recovery services, legislation, and opioid overdose prevention training.

INTRODUCTION

In the United States, opioid overdose continues to affect thousands each year. The Center for Disease Control and Prevention (CDC, 2020) estimates that nearly 841,000 people have died from a drug overdose since 1999.[1] In recent years, the opioid death rate has been exacerbated by synthetic opioids, most notably illicit fentanyl and heroin. In 2015, in the recognition of this national epidemic, President Obama issued a federal memorandum as well as announced federal, state, local, and private sector efforts aimed at addressing heroin use and prescription drug misuse with a focus on opioid prescriber training and improving access to addiction treatment. The US Department of Health and Human Services (HHS, 2015) followed suit and prioritized addressing opioid abuse, focusing on implementing evidence-based approaches to reduce opioid overdoses and the prevalence of opioid use disorder (OUD).[2] Subsequently, in response to continued increases in opioid-related morbidity and mortality, in 2017, HHS declared a nationwide public health emergency

New York University, Rory Meyers College of Nursing, 433 First room 420 Avenue, New York, NY 10010, USA
E-mail address: Sg141@nyu.edu

Nurs Clin N Am 57 (2022) 477–488
https://doi.org/10.1016/j.cnur.2022.04.013

regarding the opioid crisis, leading to the development of a 5-point harm reduction strategy.[3] Nurses can be instrumental in educating patients, families, and community members about ways to combat this epidemic, instrumental in advocating for reform, as well as continue to bring awareness to this health crisis and provoke dialogue about ongoing solutions to end it.

Scope of the Problem

In 2019, 70,630 drug overdose deaths occurred in the United States, with nearly 50,000 (70%) of those deaths involving an opioid. Opioid overdose deaths, including prescription opioids, heroin, and synthetic opioids like fentanyl have increased over 6-fold since 1999.[1,4] In recent years, increases in opioid prescriptions such as morphine, Percocet, and Oxycontin have been a major factor in opioid addiction or accidental overdose; however, there has been recent surges in illicit opioid-related overdose deaths, driven largely by heroin and fentanyl.[4–8] (**Box 2**) While more than 14,000 (28%) opioid overdose deaths involved prescription opioids in 2019, there was a nearly 7% decrease from 2018 to 2019. According to the 2019 National Survey on Drug Use and Health (NSDUH, 2020), 9.3 million people misused opioids in the past year, with the majority misusing prescription pain relievers.[9] While the most common reason among past year misusers was for pain relief (65.7%), others included to feel good or get high (11.3%) and to relax and relieve tension (10%). Assistance with sleep (3.7%), helping with feelings or emotions (3.8%), and to experiment or see what the drug was like (2.2%) were less common.[9] There are several factors that increase the risk for opioid misuse (**Box 3**) The rate of overdose deaths involving synthetic opioids was more than 11 times higher in 2019 than in 2013.[9] With synthetic opioids such as fentanyl being the main driver of this major public health concern, rates were highest among adults age 35 to 44 in 2019.[1,2] Approximately one-third of all opioid deaths in 2019 involved heroin. Cocaine was involved in nearly 1 in 5 overdose deaths.[1,10] In recent years, the drug death rate is rising most steeply among African Americans nationally, with many falling victims to fentanyl.[1,2,9]

The COVID-19 pandemic, marked by social isolation and mental health concerns, financial crisis, and changes in care delivery due to shut-downs, has had a huge impact on opioid overdose morbidity and mortality in the United States, leading to the most significant 1-year increase in drug overdose deaths in the last 30 years. From 2019 to 2020, the US saw drug overdose rate increases for all sexes, ages, ethnicities, and Hispanic-origin groups. In 2020, over 91,000 drug overdose deaths occurred in the US, 31% higher than the rate in 2019 (21.6–28.3).[4] To put that into perspective, that's enough to fill the NY Giant's Football Stadium. Rates remained highest among people aged 35 to 44. The rate of overdose deaths involving drugs including fentanyl, fentanyl analogs, and tramadol increased by 56% from 2019 to 2020 (11.4–17.8). While the rates of overdose deaths involving natural and semisynthetic opioids, including drugs such as oxycodone and hydrocodone, decreased between 2017 and 2019, increases were noted in 2020. While overdose death involving heroin decreased, cocaine death rates increased in 2020, with rates 50% higher than 2019.[4,8,10]

Definitions

Box 1.

Opioid Basics

When opioids are taken, they attach to opioid receptors on nerve cells in the brain, spinal cord, gut, and other parts of the body, subsequently blocking pain messages sent

Box 1
Key terms

Tolerance	Diminished response to a substance because of repeated use leading to the individual's need for increased amounts of a substance to get the same effect.
Dependence	The body has adapted to the presence of a substance, precipitating withdrawal symptoms if the substance is no longer used.
Addiction	Chronic disease characterized by compulsive drug seeking and use, despite harmful consequences.
Drug misuse	The use of illegal drugs and/or the use of one's own prescription drugs in a manner other than as directed by the prescriber (ie, in greater amounts, more often, or longer amount of time). Also includes using someone else's prescription.
Drug poisoning/Overdose	Harm that results from unintentional or intentional intake of a substance.
Illicit drugs	Nonmedical use of a variety of drugs that are prohibited by law, including but not limited to amphetamine-type stimulants, marijuana/cannabis, cocaine, heroin, other opioids, and synthetic drugs, such as illicitly manufactured fentanyl and ecstasy.
Opioids	Natural, synthetic, or semi-synthetic chemicals that interact with opioid receptors on nerve cells in the body and brain, reducing the intensity of pain signals and feelings of pain
Natural and semisynthetic opioids	Includes drugs such as morphine, codeine, hydrocodone, oxymorphone, and oxycodone.
Synthetic opioids	Includes drugs such as methadone, fentanyl, fentanyl analogs, and tramadol.

Data from Refs.[5,7,11–13]

from the body through the spinal cord to the brain. This reduces the intensity of pain signals and feelings of pain. In addition, the drug affects the brain's "reward center," leading to surges in feel-good neurotransmitters such as dopamine resulting in euphoria ("high"). This response serves as the reinforcement of the pleasurable but unhealthy behavior of taking the substance, which can lead an individual to repeat the behavior.[11–13] Side effects of opioids can include sleepiness, constipation, and nausea. Opioids can also cause more serious side effects that can be life-threatening, such as shallow breathing, bradycardia, and loss of consciousness.[11–14]
Box 2

Over time, opioids can make the individual's brain and body believe the drug is necessary for survival. With repeated drug use, the body can become tolerant, as the brain adapts to reward center stimulation.[11,13,15] Because of the reduction in

Box 2
Most common drugs involved in prescription opioid overdose deaths

- Methadone
- Oxycodone
- Hydrocodone

Data from Refs.[4,7,10]

euphoria that occurs, the body requires an increased quantity of the drug to produce the same high the individual felt when first taking the drug. An individual can also become physically dependent on the opioid, resulting in withdrawal symptoms (agitation, anxiety, sweating, muscle aches) if the drug is not taken.[11,13,15]

Addiction is a chronic disease and complex condition whereby repeated drug use can lead to brain changes that challenge an individual's self-control and interfere with their ability to resist intense urges to take drugs.[11,13,15] Brain chemical changes related to long-term drug use can affect learning, judgment, decision-making, memory, and behavior. Addiction is characterized by compulsive, or difficult to control, drug-seeking behavior, despite the harmful consequences.[13,15] The brain changes that occur with addiction can be persistent, thus relapse can occur, whereby people in recovery are at increased risk for returning to drug use even after years of not taking the drug. As with other chronic health conditions, addiction treatment is individualized, ongoing, reviewed often, and adjusted based on the individual's response and needs. Effective treatment options include inpatient detox, inpatient rehab, medication-assisted treatment (MAT), cognitive behavioral therapy, individual and group counseling, and 12-step programs.[13,15] MAT in combination with counseling and behavioral therapies, is not only useful in the treatment of OUD, but can also prevent or reduce opioid overdose. The 3 FDA-approved medications to treat OUDs include naltrexone, buprenorphine, and methadone.[13,15,16] Methadone, often appropriate for patients with histories of heavy and problematic opioid use, is an opioid agonist that occupies and activates opioid receptors, eliminating withdrawal symptoms and relieving drug cravings without producing euphoria. Similarly, buprenorphine, a partial opioid agonist, binds to those same opioid receptors but activates them less strongly than full agonists do. Like methadone, it can reduce cravings and withdrawal symptoms in a person with an OUD without producing euphoria.[13,15,16] Evidence supports buprenorphine therapy to help stop the illicit use of opioids and increase treatment retention.[16] Research has found buprenorphine to be similarly effective as methadone for treating OUDs, as long as it is given at a sufficient dose and for sufficient duration.[13,15,16]

Primary prevention strategies, like illicit substance use screening, are important and should be conducted for all patients in all settings.[14] The NIDA Quick Screen is a useful tool appropriate for patients 18 or older. The tool, found to be 100% sensitive and 75.3% specific for the detection of a substance use disorder, was adapted from a single screener question used in primary care by Smith and colleagues.[17] With this tool, the health care provider can easily and quickly gather information regarding frequency of substance use (including alcohol) over the last year. It can be used as a conversation starter to gauge substance use and allow for appropriate brief interventions and referral to specialist care as needed based on the findings.[13,17] **Box 3**

Opioid overdose can occur due to many factors, such as deliberate (overmedicating) or unintentional (miscalculated dose, misunderstanding dosing instructions) misuse of a prescription, or illicit use of an opioid (such as heroin)[11,14] It can also occur if an individual uses an opioid or other unknown drug that may have been contaminated with other potent opioids such as fentanyl, which is 50 to 100 times stronger than morphine and 30 to 50 times stronger than heroin[11–13] Overdose can also occur when opioids are taken in conjunction with alcohol, other illicit drugs, or with other medications such as benzodiazepines or other psychotropic medications that are used in the treatment of mental disorders. Individuals who use opioids in combination with these substances are particularly at risk for overdose as all of these substances can cause respiratory depression. The life-threatening effects of opioid overdose,

Box 3
Risk factors for opioid misuse

- Unemployment
- Living in rural areas and having low income
- Family history of substance abuse
- Young age
- Heavy tobacco use
- Taking high daily dosages of prescription pain relievers
- Obtaining overlapping prescriptions from multiple providers and pharmacies
- History of severe depression or anxiety
- History of alcohol or other substance use disorders
- History of criminal activity or legal problems including DUIs
- Regular contact with high-risk people or high-risk environments
- Risk-taking or thrill-seeking behavior

Data from Refs.[11–13]

including shallow breathing, bradycardia, and loss of consciousness, can lead to death in a matter of minutes[11–14] **Box 4**

ROLE OF THE PROFESSIONAL NURSE

The ever-worsening opioid overdose epidemic requires urgent action and an all-hands-on-deck approach. It will take a comprehensive and coordinated approach from all members of the health care team and health care institutions, in addition to

Box 4
Risk factors for opioid overdose

Changes in tolerance	Individuals who have intentionally or unintentionally abstained from drug use for any reason, including inconsistent access to drugs (ie, hospitalization, incarceration, detox, rehab, covid isolation, are at increased risk of an overdose. When an individual has not used a substance for a period of time, tolerance decreases. As a result, when attempting to take the amount of a substance they took prior to abstaining, they can overdose.
Mixing drugs	Research shows that most drug overdoses involve more than one substance, including alcohol or other central nervous system (CNS) depressants such as benzodiazepines. Mixing substances can increase san individuals' risk of experiencing an overdose.
Drug quality	The strength and purity of drugs purchased illicitly (off the street or online) are unknown. Unpredictable changes in drug quality, purity, and strength may occur and can lead to overdose.
Previous nonfatal overdose	Previous experience with a nonfatal overdose places an individual at higher risk of experiencing another overdose.
Using alone	Using alone is a risk factor for a fatal overdose because there is no one present to respond, to call 911, or to administer naloxone in the event that an individual overdoses.

Data from Refs.[12,13]

governmental officials, public safety, and community organizations. The 2017 HHS opioid overdose public health crisis declaration included a 5-point strategy. This comprehensive strategy incorporated improving access to addiction prevention, treatment, and recovery support services; targeting the availability and distribution of overdose-reversing drugs such as naloxone; strengthening public health data reporting and collection; supporting cutting-edge research on addiction and pain; and advancing the practice of pain management.[3] Health care professionals play an important role in combatting this major public health problem by incorporating innovative and established evidenced-based prevention and response strategies. Nurses, as members of the health care team, are uniquely positioned as direct patient care providers, patient educators, patient advocates, and leaders to play a critical role in these efforts.

Effective Pain Management and Education

One of the HHS's 5 major priorities in combatting the opioid epidemic is advancing better practices for pain management.[3] Pain management is essential for improving the quality of life of patients with acute and chronic pain. When patients do not have adequate pain control, they may resort to other methods, like illicit substances. In 2010, compelled by HHS and the National Institute of Health (NIH), the Institute of Medicine (IOM) convened an ad hoc committee that included a diverse group of experts to conduct a study and make recommendations regarding pain as a significant health problem in the United States. This resulted in the IOM report, *Relieving pain in America: A blueprint for transforming prevention, care, education, and research, barriers occur at the system, clinician, patient, and insurance levels.*[18] Later, the IOM report guided the development of the National Pain Strategy, with an aim of reducing the burden of pain and its associated morbidity and disability across the lifespan.[19] One of the main objectives of this strategy is pain prevention and care. Nurses are at the forefront and are well equipped to assess pain and the need for pharmacologic and nonpharmacologic pain interventions, ensure that adequate pain relief measures are implemented, and advocate for those in pain.

Pain is cited as the most common reason Americans access the health care system, with chronic pain as the most common cause of long-term disability.[18–20] In 2019, approximately 20% of US adults had chronic pain and 7% had high-impact chronic pain (pain that frequently limited their life or work activities).[20] Not only does ineffective pain management have a huge impact on quality of life, but it can lead to emotional distress, functional limitations, problems in initiating and maintaining sleep, changes in appetite, social isolation, depression, increases financial burdens, caregiving burdens, and altered coping.[21,22]

Having basic knowledge about pain, including diagnosis, treatment, complications, and prognosis, other available treatment options, and information about over-the-counter medications and self-help strategies is critical for nurses. A timely and thorough physical examination, including the use of culturally appropriate pain scales and assessment of nonverbal pain behaviors is key. Nurses should thoroughly assess pain and communicate their findings with the other members of the health care team to ensure the initiation of adequate person-centered pain relief measures, as well as evaluate effectiveness of interventions. Nurses must advocate for those in pain and focus on prevention or control of pain, not waiting for severe pain to occur before treating it.

Managing pain can be challenging. Pain is often multifactorial and, as such, warrants a multimodal approach to treatment, using both pharmacologic and nonpharmacological approaches. Pharmacologic treatment options can include a variety of medications, including but not limited to NSAIDS, topical preparations, muscle relaxers, and opioids.[23,24] While opioids are appropriate and often used for moderate to severe pain, both nociceptive and neuropathic pain, unfortunately, increases in opioid prescriptions such as morphine and oxycodone, has been a major factor in opioid addiction or accidental overdose.[4–8] Research shows that most people who are addicted to opioids took their first opioid from a relative or friend to whom it was legitimately prescribed.[9] Pain medications can have an impact on medical conditions and/or medications. Nonpharmacological strategies such as massage, relaxation/meditation, TENS unit, physical or occupational therapy, chiropractic treatments, acupuncture, exercise, and physical modalities (heat, cold) can reduce the number of medications needed to treat pain. It is well understood that pain is also influenced by cognition, affect, and behavior; therefore, other therapies such as cognitive behavioral therapy and mind-body conditioning practices such as yoga, tai chi, qigong can be beneficial.[25] (**Fig 1**) The health care team must ensure that patients and their families are provided with information and understand the risks and benefits of pain treatment options, and in addition be supportive of patient pain self-management strategies.[23–25] It is important to note that cultural background and beliefs have a role in how patients interpret, express, manage pain, and make pain or palliative care decision; therefore, other treatment options may include the use of spiritual healers, herbs, coining, and cupping to name a few.[26] **Box 5**

Overdose Prevention, Recognition, and Treatment

Not only do nurses play a role in pain assessment and management, including patient education on the proper use of opioids, but they are also instrumental in implementing other measures to prevent fatal overdose, including educating patients and their families about opioid overdose signs/symptoms and a plan of action should any of these occur. Nurses should look out for and ensure that their patients and family members are familiar with opioid overdose signs/symptoms, such as unresponsiveness, pinpoint pupils, decrease in respirations or nosey breathing, cold and clammy skin, and cyanotic nails and lips.[11,12] Nurses should become familiar with the many local and federal initiatives to combat opioid misuse and overdose including conducting surveillance and research, better addiction treatment and recovery services,

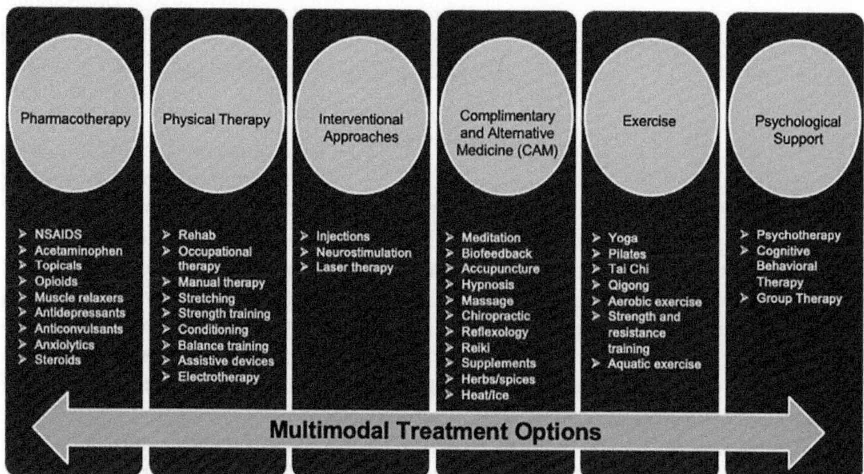

Fig. 1. Multimodal treatment options.

Box 5
Pain management pearls

Timely, thorough assessment	• Scales: Faces, Numeric, Visual Analog, PAINAD • Pain history: onset, location, duration, intensity, characteristics, and aggravating and palliating factors • Nonverbal behaviors: facial expressions, vocalizations, body language/movements, changes in interpersonal interactions, changes in mental status changes in usual activity • Psychological screening: depression, anxiety, and substance use screening • Assess social networks and family involvement • Beware of red flags: pain that awakens the patient, neurologic deficits, cold, pale, or cyanotic limb, new bowel/bladder dysfunction, severe abdominal pain, signs of shock • Rule out other causative pathologies (ie, urinary retention, constipation, infection) • Ensure basic comfort needs are being met (hunger, toileting, loneliness, fear)
Ensure the initiation of adequate pain relief measures	• Risk or prescription opioid abuse assessment tools: Opioid Risk Tool, SOAPP • Scheduling – focus on prevention or control, around the clock for constant pain, fast-acting drugs for breakthrough pain, do not wait until pain is severe before intervening • Time to effectiveness varies by route/formulation - pill, lozenge, lollipops, spray, rectal, nasal, IV push, topical cream or patch, implantable pump, PCA • Evaluate the effectiveness of interventions - dose adjustment based on the assessment of analgesic effect vs side effects; use the smallest dose to provide effective pain control with fewest side effects
Patient and family education	• Proper use of pain medications • Proper opioid storage and titration • Recognizing and responding to potential opioid overdose

Data from Refs.[18,19,23–25]

legislation, and opioid overdose prevention training. Most importantly, nurses should be trained in the use of naloxone to treat opioid overdose (**Fig 2**) Naloxone, a lifesaving overdose medication, is an opioid antagonist that blocks the effects of opioids, immediately reversing their action· Given the first sign of overdose, naloxone works within 1 to 5 minutes.[12,13] Many local and federal initiatives are already in place to make naloxone overdose kits and training programs available.

Substance use screening with tools such as the NIDA *Quick Screen* is vital in appropriately identifying patients with or at risk for substance use disorders and ensuring the appropriate interventions and specialist referrals are made. Patients

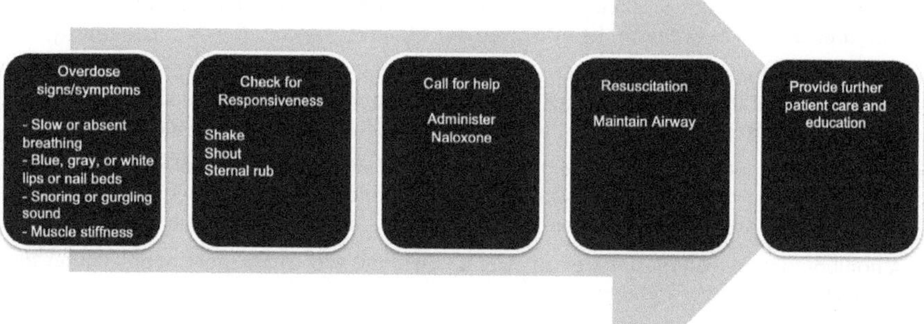

Fig. 2. Recognizing and responding to an overdose.

undergoing MAT with methadone or buprenorphine will likely continue their treatment when hospitalized, as determined by their health care providers. All patients should be educated about tolerance, dependence, and risk for misuse and overdose on an ongoing basis, reinforcing at discharge.[11,12,15] Individuals who use opioids and are not receiving opioid-based medication-assisted therapies are at greater risk of overdose, thus a naloxone kit should always be part of the patient treatment plan.[27,28]

Unfortunately, drug-related stigma still exists and has critical real-life consequences. Negative attitudes of health professionals toward patients with substance use disorders can contribute to suboptimal health care for these patients.[29] Nurses and other members of the health care team must be sure to approach patients in a nonjudgmental manor, ensuring that their own personal values and beliefs do not interfere with their ability to provide care for their patients. Negative terminology surrounding substance use disorders reinforces these barriers that prevent individuals from seeking help. Therefore, a nonjudgmental, compassionate approach should be taken to increase dialogue and create more opportunities for engagement, support, and understanding. Avoid using words that convey judgment or reinforce stigma and like abuser, addict, drug habit, junkie, staying clean, or drug seeking.[29]

SUMMARY

Opioid overdose continues to take thousands of lives each year in the United States. To reverse this epidemic, we need to not only improve the way we treat pain, but also implement effective evidence-based measures that prevent misuse, addiction, and overdose. Local and federal initiatives are in place that focuses on the HHS 5-point harm reduction strategy. Nurses as advocates can join in on the efforts of their local government or community organizations to combat the opioid epidemic advocating for expanded naloxone distribution, improved access to substance use disorder treatment, and the expansion of other harm reduction services including partnering with public safety and educating the public about the dangers of hidden fentanyl in street drugs. Nurses can be instrumental in educating patients, families, and community members about ways to combat this epidemic, instrumental in advocating for reform, as well as continuing to bring awareness to this health crisis and provoke dialogue about ongoing solutions to end it.

CLINICS CARE POINTS

- Nurses should thoroughly assess pain and communicate their findings with the other members of the health care team and ensure the initiation of adequate pain relief measures, as well as evaluate the effectiveness of interventions.
- Nonpharmacological strategies such as massage, relaxation/meditation, TENS unit, physical or occupational therapy, chiropractic treatments, acupuncture, exercise, and physical modalities (heat, cold) can reduce the number of medications needed to treat pain.
- Nurses should look out for and sure that their patients and family members are familiar with opioid overdose signs/symptoms, such as unresponsiveness, pinpoint pupils, decrease in respirations or nosey breathing, cold and clammy skin, and cyanotic nails and lips.
- A nonjudgmental, compassionate can increase dialogue and create more opportunities for engagement, support, and understanding.

CONFLICT OF INTEREST STATEMENT

The author declares that the article was conducted in the absence of any commercial or financial relationships that could be construed as a potential conflict of interest.

DISCLOSURE

The author has nothing to disclose.

REFERENCES

1. Centers for Disease Control and Prevention National Center for Health Statistics. Wide-ranging online data for epidemiologic research (WONDER). 2020. Available at: http://wonder.cdc.gov. Accessed December 12, 2021.
2. U.S. Department of Health and Human Services. Opioid abuse in the U.S. and HHS actions to address opioid-drug related overdoses and deaths. 2015. Available at: https://aspe.hhs.gov/basic-report/opioid-abuse-us-and-hhs-actions-address-opioid-drug-related-overdoses-and-deaths. Accessed December 2, 2021.
3. U.S. Department of Health and Human Services. 5-Point strategy to combat the opioid crisis. 2018. Available at: https://www.hhs.gov/opioids/about-the-epidemic/hhs-response/index.html. Accessed December 2, 2021.
4. Hedegaard H, Miniño AM, Spencer MR, et al. Drug overdose deaths in the United States, 1999–2020. NCHS Data Brief, no 428. Hyattsville, MD: National Center for Health Statistics; 2021. https://doi.org/10.15620/cdc:112340.
5. U.S. Department of Health and Human Services. What is the U.S. opioid epidemic?. 2019. Available at: https://www.hhs.gov/opioids/about-the-epidemic/index.html. Accessed November 21, 2021.
6. Centers for Disease Control and Prevention. Increases in drug and opioid overdose deaths — United States, 2000–2014. 2016. Available at. https://www.cdc.gov/mmwr/preview/mmwrhtml/mm6450a3.htm?s_cid=mm6450a3_w. Accessed December 1, 2021.
7. Centers for Disease Control and Prevention. Prescription opioids. 2017. Available at: https://www.cdc.gov/drugoverdose/opioids/prescribed.html. Accessed December 5, 2021.
8. Centers for Disease Control and Prevention. Drug overdose deaths. 2018. Available at: https://www.cdc.gov/drugoverdose/data/statedeaths.html. Accessed December 5, 2021.

9. Substance Abuse and Mental Health Services Administration. Key substance use and mental health indicators in the United States: results from the 2019 national survey on drug use and health. 2020. HHS Publication No. PEP20-07-01-001, NSDUH Series H-55). Rockville, MD: Center for Behavioral Health Statistics and Quality, Substance Abuse and Mental Health Services Administration. Available at: https://www.samhsa.gov/data/external icon. Accessed November 21, 2021.
10. Mattson CL, Tanz LJ, Quinn K, et al. Trends and geographic patterns in drug and synthetic opioid overdose deaths — United States, 2013–2019. MMWR Morb Mortal Wkly Rep 2021;70:202–7.
11. American Society of Anesthesiologists. Opioid Abuse. 2021. Available at: https://www.asahq.org/madeforthismoment/pain-management/opioid-treatment/what-are-opioids/. Accessed December 12, 2021.
12. Galanter M, Kleber H, Brady K. The American psychiatric publishing textbook of substance abuse treatment. Washington, DC: American Psychiatric Publishing; 2015.
13. American Psychiatric Association. Addiction and substance use disorder. 2021. Available at: https://www.psychiatry.org/patients-families/addiction/what-is-addiction. Accessed December 2, 2021.
14. U.S. Department of Health and Human Services. Office of the surgeon general, facing addiction in america: the surgeon general's report on alcohol, drugs, and health. Washington. 2016. Available at: https://addiction.surgeongeneral.gov/sites/default/files/surgeon-generals-report.pdf. Accessed December 2, 2021.
15. Bart G. Maintenance medication for opiate addiction: the foundation of recovery. J Addict Dis 2012;31(3):207–25.
16. Mattick RP, Breen C, Kimber J, et al. Buprenorphine maintenance versus placebo or methadone maintenance for opioid dependence. Cochrane Database Syst Rev 2014–;2:CD002207. Available at: https://doi.org/10.1002/14651858.CD002207.pub4. Accessed December 12, 2021.
17. Smith PC, Schmidt SM, Allensworth-Davies D, et al. A single-question screening test for drug use in primary care. Arch Intern Med 2010;170(13):1155–60.
18. Institute of Medicine (US). Committee on advancing pain research, care, and education. relieving pain in America: a blueprint for transforming prevention, care, education, and research. Washington (DC): National Academies Press (US); 2011. PMID: 22553896. Available at: https://pubmed.ncbi.nlm.nih.gov/22553896/.
19. U.S. Department of Health and Human Services, National Institutes of Health. Interagency pain research coordinating committee. national pain strategy: a comprehensive population health-level strategy for pain. 2016. Available at: https://iprcc.nih.gov/sites/default/files/HHSNational_Pain_Strategy_508C.pdf. Accessed December 12, 2021.
20. Zelaya CE, Dahlhamer JM, Lucas JW, et al. Chronic pain and high-impact chronic pain among U.S. adults, 2019. NCHS Data Brief, no 390. Hyattsville, MD: National Center for Health Statistics; 2020.
21. Artner J, Cakir B, Spiekermann JA, et al. Prevalence of sleep deprivation in patients with chronic neck and back pain: a retrospective evaluation of 1016 patients. J Pain Res 2013;6:1–6.
22. Chen Q, Hayman L, Shmerling R, et al. Characteristics of Chronic pain associated with sleep difficulty in older adults: The Maintenance of balance,

independent living, intellect, and zest in the elderly (MOBILIZE) Boston Study. J Am Geriatr Soc 2011;59(8):1385–92.
23. Krebs EE, Gravely A, Nugent S, et al. Effect of opioid vs nonopioid medications on pain-related function in patients with chronic back pain or hip or knee osteoarthritis pain: the SPACE randomized clinical trial. JAMA 2018;319(9):872–82. https://doi.org/10.1001/jama.2018.0899.
24. Dowell D, Haegerich TM, Chou R. CDC guideline for prescribing opioids for chronic pain — United States, 2016. MMWR Recomm Rep 2016;65(1):1–49. https://doi.org/10.15585/mmwr.rr6501e1external icon.
25. Skelly AC, Chou R, Dettori JR, et al. Noninvasive nonpharmacological treatment for chronic pain: a systematic review update. Rockville, MD: Agency for Healthcare Research and Quality 2020. https://doi.org/10.23970/AHRQEPCCER227. Comparative effectiveness review no. 227. (prepared by the pacific northwest evidence-based practice center under contract No. 290-2015-00009-I.) AHRQ Publication No. 20-EHC009.
26. Givler A, Bhatt H, Maani-Fogelman PA. The importance of cultural competence in pain and palliative care. Treasure Island (FL): StatPearls Publishing; 2021. Available at: https://www.ncbi.nlm.nih.gov/books/NBK493154/.
27. Betts KS, Chan G, Mcilwraith F, et al. Differences in polysubstance use patterns and drug-related outcomes between people who inject drugs receiving and not receiving opioid substitution therapies. Addiction 2016;111. https://doi.org/10.1111/add.13339.
28. Walley AY, Xuan Z, Hackman HH, et al. Opioid overdose rates and implementation of overdose education and nasal naloxone distribution in Massachusetts: interrupted time series analysis. BMJ 2013;346:f174.
29. van Boekel LC, Brouwers EP, van Weeghel J, et al. Stigma among health professionals towards patients with substance use disorders and its consequences for healthcare delivery: systematic review. Drug and Alcohol Dependence 2013;131(1–2):23–35.

Racial and Ethnic Disparities in Autism Spectrum Disorder

Implications for Care

Susan Brasher, PhD, RN, CPNP-PC, FAAN[a,*],
Jennifer L. Stapel-Wax, PsyD[b],
Lisa Muirhead, DNP, APRN, ANP-BC, FAANP, FAAN[a]

KEYWORDS

- Autism • Autism spectrum disorder • Health care disparities
- Vulnerable populations • Racial and ethnic disparities

KEY POINTS

- Autism spectrum disorder (ASD) is a neurodevelopmental condition that emerges in early childhood and spans the lifespan.
- Racial and ethnic disparities among individuals with ASD contribute to health inequities and poorer outcomes.
- Misconceptions of ASD alongside racial and ethnic biases have serious health implications.
- Youth and adults from marginalized groups with ASD are at increased risk of being misunderstood during health care and law enforcement encounters.

INTRODUCTION

Autism spectrum disorder (ASD) is a complex neurodevelopmental disorder characterized by core symptoms inclusive of difficulties with social interaction and communication, as well as the presence of restrictive, repetitive behavior.[1] Symptoms of ASD appear early in childhood and persist into adulthood. In addition to the core symptoms, individuals with ASD also experience several co-occurring medical and psychiatric conditions.[2] Research suggests that greater than 95% of individuals with ASD experience at least one of the following co-occurring conditions: neurologic disorders (eg, seizures), gastrointestinal disorders (eg, feeding difficulties, diarrhea,

[a] Nell Hodgson Woodruff School of Nursing, Emory University, 1520 Clifton Road, Atlanta, GA 30322, USA; [b] Division of Autism and Related Disorders, Department of Pediatrics, Emory University School of Medicine, Infant Toddler Clinical Research Operations, Infant Toddler Community Outreach Research Core, Marcus Autism Center, Children's Healthcare of Atlanta, 1920 Briarcliff Road, Atlanta, GA 30329, USA
* Corresponding author.
E-mail address: susan.n.brasher@emory.edu

Nurs Clin N Am 57 (2022) 489–499
https://doi.org/10.1016/j.cnur.2022.04.014
0029-6465/22/

constipation), sleep disorders, depression, anxiety, bipolar disorder, attention deficit hyperactivity disorder, and behavioral challenges.[3] As a result, individuals with ASD have significantly higher health care utilization rates across Emergency Department,[4,5] Primary Care, Mental Health, and Laboratory settings.[6] Individuals with ASD require substantial support to address the myriad of co-occurring conditions that are complicated by the developmental impairments associated with ASD. Yet, studies have found that despite the overwhelming increase in health care needs, individuals with ASD are more likely to have unmet needs in terms of receiving necessary services[7]; this discordance represents a growing health care crisis. Therefore, the purpose of this paper is to provide an overview of ASD and racial and ethnic disparities that contribute to unmet health care needs, as well as recommendations for change.

Currently, 1 in 44 children are diagnosed with ASD.[8] As children with ASD transition into adulthood, an increased prevalence of ASD has been estimated in 5,437,988 (2.1%) of the adult US population.[9] Evidence demonstrates early ASD diagnosis and access to services improves long-term developmental outcomes.[10–12] Yet, for some children the ASD diagnosis comes much later and access to services is not equitable.[13–15] These delays in care have lifelong consequences.

Despite the increasing prevalence of ASD,[16] disparities exist among specific groups (eg, racial, ethnic, cultural, socioeconomic, geographic, gender, sexual identity), thus creating disproportionately poorer outcomes.[17–21] Individuals with ASD who are disadvantaged by disparities experience increased morbidity and decreased life expectancy compared with both the general population and individuals with ASD who do not encounter these disparities.[17] Greater awareness is required by nurses and other health care providers on the impact that these disparities have on health and health outcomes, as well as ways to improve health care encounters for individuals with ASD.

DISPARITIES IN AUTISM SPECTRUM DISORDER

Disparities exist when health outcomes are seen to be greater or lesser between populations.[22] Racial and ethnic disparities among the general population are a result of significant differences in access to needed services, health status, and health outcomes.[23,24] These differences are magnified in individuals with ASD who frequently experience unmet health care needs and poorer health outcomes across the lifespan.[17,25–27]Among racial and ethnic minority groups, significant disparities have been noted to affect access to timely ASD diagnosis,[14,15] health and education services,[26,27] and autism-related services.[14,19]

Racial Disparities and Autism Spectrum Disorder

Although ASD occurs across all racial and ethnic groups, disparities disproportionately affect specific racial groups (ie, Black) and ethnic groups (ie, Hispanic or LatinX). Comparatively, White children are more likely to be diagnosed with ASD earlier in childhood than Black and Hispanic or LatinX children, thus affecting earlier interventions through health and education services for behavioral modification; training for social skill development; speech, physical, and occupational therapies; and cognitive-based therapies.[27] Research indicates that Black children are more likely to have a misdiagnosis and delayed ASD diagnosis, representing an approximate 1.5-year delay compared with children of other races.[28] Specifically, when compared with White children, Black children are diagnosed 1.6 years later, have 2.6 greater odds of incorrect diagnosis, are 5.1 times more likely to be misdiagnosed with adjustment disorder, incur 2.4 greater odds of being diagnosed with conduct disorder, and are more likely hospitalized in psychiatric units.[25] Of great concern is the 3-year delay between the time when parents of Black children reported concerns to a health care provider to the time when their child received an ASD diagnosis.[19] These delays can be attributed to structural and systemic racism.[29] In addition, recent research noted Black children with ASD to be significantly more likely to have an intellectual disability compared with White or Hispanic or LatinX children with ASD.[13] The presence of intellectual disability in 49.8% of Black children diagnosed with ASD is alarmingly high compared with White and Hispanic or LatinX children, highlighting the sizable impact racial and ethnic disparities have on cognitive impairment as a result of delayed ASD diagnosis and access to services.[30]

Ethnic Disparities and Autism Sprectrum Disorder

Ethnic disparities in ASD diagnosis and inequitable access to services have also been cited throughout the literature.[18,20,30,31] Barriers to ASD identification and access to services in the Hispanic or LatinX population are abundant and include provider discrimination,[32] stigma, lack of access to health care services due to noncitizenship or low income, and non-English primary language.[30] As a result, Hispanic or LatinX children are less likely to be diagnosed with ASD compared with White and Black children.[13] Subsequently, Hispanic or LatinX children with ASD are more likely than White children to have lower IQ scores (ie, IQ < 70).[13] This delay in diagnosis and consequential poor cognitive outcomes once again highlight the impact ethnic disparities have on ASD identification and access to services. Studies also suggest that Hispanic or LatinX individuals are less likely to have usual sources of primary care, and have lower health care use, including mental health care, compared with Black and White individuals.[24] Combined with limited English language proficiency, these factors may present additional unique challenges for Hispanic or LatinX families navigating systems.[27]

Racial and Ethnic Disparate Outcomes Among Youth and Adults with Autism Spectrum Disorder

Racial and ethnic disparities in ASD, combined with other disadvantaging factors, significantly influence the ability to access quality health systems and adequate care.[17] Studies have found that Black and Hispanic or LatinX youth and young adults with ASD experience greater adversities when encountering health care systems.[17,19] These differences in quality access and care have resulted in disparate psychiatric and physical health outcomes.

When compared with the general population, research suggests that adults with ASD have higher rates of physical health conditions, including hypertension, diabetes, epilepsy, skin disorder, and endocrine disorders.[33–35] Other studies indicate that more than half of the adults with ASD (54%) have a psychiatric condition, indicating the risk of psychiatric disorders in adults with ASD is significantly increased, ranging from 2.9 times higher for depression to 22 times higher for schizophrenia, compared with the general population.[34] These findings indicate increased health care needs and service utilization. Yet, studies have found a higher proportion of unmet needs in terms of services and access to providers among individuals with ASD.[7]

In examining ethnic and racial differences in physical health conditions among adults with ASD, studies have found Hispanic or LatinX adults had higher odds of obesity, diabetes, hepatic disorders, hypertension, vision deficits and blindness, headaches, and cardiovascular disease.[33] Similarly, Black adults with ASD had higher odds of hypertension, diabetes, obesity, asthma, and hospitalization for cardiovascular disease compared with White adults with ASD.[33] Considering the increase in chronic medical conditions among these racial and ethnic minority groups with ASD, access to health care services is critical to improve health and health outcomes.

Racial and ethnic disparities have also been found to exist in psychiatric conditions among adults with ASD, indicating Black and Hispanic or LatinX individuals have higher rates of psychiatric diagnoses (eg, schizophrenia) and additional higher rates of drug abuse or dependence among Black individuals with ASD. Researchers note that these disparate conditions may reflect inequities in access to quality mental health care for Black and Hispanic or LatinX adults with ASD.[33]

Risk Associated with Law Enforcement Encounters

Of special concern are the risk and vulnerabilities among adults with ASD and encounters with law enforcement officers (LEO) and the impact these have on their health. Many LEO lack adequate training in recognizing symptoms and characteristics of ASD[36] and may misinterpret certain behaviors and actions, such as avoidance of eye contact, difficulty with social communication, repetitive behaviors (eg, rocking back and forth), and attempts to leave the scene, as suspicious, threatening, disorderly, or lacking compliance.[36–38] These encounters with individuals with ASD have resulted in excessive use of force[36] and resulted in physical and psychological harm or even death in some instances. Researchers report that by the age of 21 years, 20% of individuals with ASD have engaged with LEOs and 5% resulted in arrest.[37,38] In the study by Gardner and Campbell (2020) involving LEOs responding to calls involving individuals with ASD, 15% of LEOs indicated use of physical force and 25% of LEOs indicated the call resulted in involuntary hospitalization.[37,38] Considering the range of core symptoms of ASD, individuals with ASD may have difficulty following LEO commands, which can elevate risk of police harm. Although issues with LEOs may affect any individual with ASD, young Black men with ASD are 7 times more likely to encounter LEOs, and when compared with White men, young Black men have 3 times the likelihood of being killed by LEOs.[39] These findings are concerning and have significant implications for health-, policy-, and competency-based education among law enforcement officers.

Implications for Nursing and Other Health Care Providers

In addition to poorer health outcomes among ethnic and racial groups,[17] individuals with ASD face poorer quality of life as a result of diminished access to assistive technologies, caregiver training, autism-related services, acceptance, and inclusion.[40] Nurses and other health care providers have the capacity to improve quality of life, health, and health outcomes of individuals with ASD. Although complex and deeply rooted, recognition of bias and the effects of structural inequalities associated with racism must be named and addressed in nursing and other health care professions. Further education and development of nurses and other health care providers, inclusive of implicit bias and cultural intelligence training, is required.

MISCONCEPTIONS OF AUTISM SPECTRUM DISORDER

Despite the growing awareness of ASD, several misconceptions exist (**Table 1**). Such misconceptions affect timely diagnosis, access to services, and receipt of quality health care. Misconceptions of ASD in racial and ethnic groups further contribute to poorer health and health outcomes. Therefore, nurses and other health care providers require specialized education and training on ASD and ways best to engage individuals from marginalized groups with ASD during health care encounters.

Table 1
Misconceptions of autism spectrum disorder

Misconception	Truth
All individuals with ASD seem the same	ASD is a heterogeneous disorder, meaning that although the core symptoms of ASD (eg, social interaction deficits, communication difficulties, repetitive behaviors) remain the same, their severity and manifestation may seem differently in individuals. This contributes to a wide spectrum of symptoms in individuals with ASD.[46]
All individuals with ASD have the same skills or difficulties	Although individuals with ASD share difficulties with the core symptoms of ASD (eg, social interaction deficits, communication difficulties, repetitive behaviors), every individual with ASD has different abilities, skills, and ways of coping with difficulties. What helps one individual with ASD to cope with a situation may not help another individual.[47]
Individuals with ASD are usually nonverbal and unable to communicate	Some individuals with ASD may have speech delay or may not use words to communicate. However, some children are extremely verbal and thus communication abilities vary widely across the spectrum. It is important to note that even if a person is unable to communicate with words, they still have the capacity, need, and right to communicate with health care professionals.[47]
All individuals with ASD have savant abilities, such as those portrayed in movies and TV shows	A small percent (10%) of individuals with ASD may exhibit savant abilities in which their skills and knowledge exceed the general population.[48] It is important to identify and appreciate the unique skills of all individuals with ASD, rather than view their characteristics through a deficit model. Movies and TV shows are not representative of everyone on the autism spectrum and can further contribute to misconceptions.
Individuals with ASD are violent and aggressive	Individuals with ASD experience altered sensory perception, which can result in sensory overload in relation to the environment (eg, lights, sounds, smell, touch). This can result in inability to cope with sensory stimulation and in emotional distress (eg, anxiety, hyperactivity) or manifest in behavioral outbursts (eg, aggression, self-injury, harm to others).[41] However, deescalating techniques and coping mechanisms can be used to avoid or minimize these situations. Individuals with ASD rarely act violently out of malice or pose a danger to society.[48]
ASD only occurs in White men	Data suggest that boys are 4.5 times more likely to be identified than girls. In addition, White children are 1.1 times more likely to be diagnosed with ASD compared with Black children and 1.2 times more common to be identified compared with Hispanic and LatinX.[30] However, these data reflect the children who are being diagnosed younger than 8-year-old and does not reflect racial and ethnic minority groups who often are undiagnosed, misdiagnosed, or later diagnosed. Similarly, girls with ASD are often undiagnosed, misdiagnosed, or later diagnosed due to misconceptions and differing or less obvious ASD signs compared with boys, which negatively affects their health and health outcomes.[49]

Table 2
Techniques to minimize traumatic experiences for individuals with autism spectrum disorder

Adjustment	Technique	Rationale
Sensory modifications	• Reduce/Dim lights • Reduce noise exposure/ Ensure patient is located away from excessive noise/ high-traffic areas (eg, nurse's station, elevator, extremely vocal patients or those in pain, front desk)	In addition to the core symptoms of ASD (eg, social interaction deficits, communication difficulties, repetitive behaviors), individuals with ASD often have strong sensory reactions to light, sound, tactile, smell and taste. These heightened sensory reactions can lead to mounting anxiety and inability to cope.
Communication modifications	1. Identify every individual's preferred communication method (eg, verbal, sign language, written, technology assistance, writing board, picture exchange card system) 2. Use clear, concise communication 3. Use visual supports as needed 4. Explain what you are doing in advance 5. Speak in a quieter tone	Individuals with ASD have varying degrees of communication abilities and preferences in which they would like to communicate. Individuals with ASD tend to be literal and concrete. Therefore, direct and clear communication should be used, without jargon or innuendos. Individuals with ASD may prefer/rely on visual supports to communicate. In addition, individuals with ASD have an insistence of sameness and thus prefer to be communicated in advance before procedures or assessments are performed. Communicating in a quieter tone can also prevent sensory overload.
Personnel modifications	• Use the minimum amount of personnel for any visit, encounter, or procedure • Schedule visits during less busy times of the day • Allow extra time during procedures, assessments, and visits	Having too many personnel during a visit, encounter, or procedure may increase anxiety and sensory overload for individuals with ASD. Individuals with ASD will be able to cope better during visits with less stimuli, which typically occurs at certain times of the day (eg, before/ after lunch, etc.). Moving quickly through procedures, assessment, or visits will likely increase anxiety in individuals with ASD.

(*continued on next page*)

Table 2
(*continued*)

Adjustment	Technique	Rationale
Preference modification	1. Document every individual's likes, dislikes, and triggers	Care of individuals with ASD should be highly customizable. Individuals with ASD have varying likes, dislikes, and triggers. Documentation of these preferences should be kept and communicated between nurses and other health care providers.

Aside from education on the misconceptions of ASD, particularly across racial and ethnic minority groups, nurses and other health care providers require training in effective ways to deliver quality patient-centered care to individuals with ASD.[41] Included in this training should be considerations for ways to minimize traumatic experiences, including the avoidance of excessive force. Incorporating these techniques (**Table 2**) can translate to improved health and health outcomes during health care encounters, particularly for racial and ethnic minority groups whose behaviors may be misattributed and result in excessive force.

DISCUSSION

Given that ASD is a life-long condition, disparate outcomes of individuals with ASD arising in childhood and continuing throughout adulthood have profound consequences for diverse racial and ethnic groups.[33,42,43] In a population with notably increased psychiatric and medical comorbidities, individuals with ASD experience greater health care utilization rates across health care settings.[4–6] Yet, health care encounters vary across the spectrum and in relation to racial and ethnic groups.

Addressing the impact of racial and ethnic disparities in the identification, diagnosis, and access to services for individuals with ASD is of paramount concern. There are multiple misperceptions and beliefs about ASD that create barriers to equitable opportunities for diagnosis and access to services. These misperceptions are more noted among Black and Hispanic or Latinx individuals with ASD, where behavioral symptoms of ASD in these populations have been attributed to a need for discipline and "boys will be boys" sentiment rather than a developmental concern.[44] Misconceptions such as these create systemic challenges that result in poorer health and health outcomes.

Access to quality health care, including routine health visits that would allow for identification of ASD and management of comorbid psychiatric and medical conditions, disproportionally affects racial and ethnic minority groups. Although great strides have been made in the last decade, it is still the case that early identification and access to services is less likely for children who are Black and Hispanic or LatinX individuals. Later ASD diagnosis means youth access ASD services later in their developmental course, thus affect the severity of their autism symptoms; this has implications not only for their developmental and cognitive outcomes but also for their health outcomes, as they encounter health care systems with more severe ASD symptoms.

Core symptoms of ASD (eg, social interaction deficits, communication difficulties, repetitive behaviors) can directly affect the health, health care encounters, and health outcomes of individuals with ASD. Nurses and other health care providers lack adequate education and training to provide quality care to individuals with ASD in the health care setting. Through enhanced education and training, nurses can play a vital role in addressing disparities and closing the gap that results in disparate outcomes.[45]

SUMMARY

Individuals with ASD are a vulnerable population that are at higher risk for medical and psychiatric comorbidities. Ethnic and racial disparities further contribute to disparate outcomes in this already vulnerable and stigmatized population. Considering the complex intersection of ASD and multiple co-occurring conditions, individuals with ASD require special health care considerations and accommodations. Yet, many nurses and other health care providers are unfamiliar with ASD and ways to connect this population to needed resources in a timely manner and mitigate the deleterious effect of delayed care. Although ASD may be growing in attention due to the heightened prevalence, many nurses and other health care providers lack specialized training on ASD and when compounded by racial and ethnic biases, may have misconceptions of how ASD symptoms manifest and intertwine with psychiatric and medical comorbidities; this represents a growing need for health care professionals to be prepared in the best ways to assess and engage individuals with ASD in the health care setting.

CLINICS CARE POINTS

- Nurses across all health care settings are likely to encounter children and adults with ASD.
- Addressing the developmental and health-related needs of individuals with ASD requires health care providers and law enforcement officers to receive specialized training on characteristics of the full spectrum of ASD.
- Recognizing racial and ethnic differences among individuals with ASD provides an opportunity for the health care community to champion equitable access to health services and resources that improve the quality of life of individuals and families from marginalized populations.
- Special techniques can be used to minimize traumatic experiences for individuals with ASD.

DISCLOSURE

All authors have no commercial or financial conflicts to disclose.

REFERENCES

1. American Psychiatric Association, Diagnostic and statistical manual of mental disorders (DSM-5). 2013. American Psychiatric Publishing 2013. Diagnostic and statistical manual of mental disorders (5th ed.). Arlington, VA
2. Davignon MN, Qian Y, Massolo M, et al. Psychiatric and medical conditions in transition-aged individuals with ASD. Pediatrics 2018;141(Suppl 4):S335–45.
3. Soke GN, Maenner MJ, Christensen D, et al. Prevalence of co-occurring medical and behavioral conditions/symptoms among 4- and 8-year-old children with autism spectrum disorder in selected areas of the United States in 2010. J Autism Dev Disord 2018;48(8):2663–76.
4. Liu G, Pearl AM, Kong L, et al. A profile on emergency department utilization in adolescents and young adults with autism spectrum disorders [published

correction appears in J Autism Dev Disord. 2017]. J Autism Dev Disord 2017;47(2):347–58.

5. Mandell DS, Candon MK, Xie M, et al. Effect of outpatient service utilization on hospitalizations and emergency visits among youths with autism spectrum disorder. Psychiatr Serv 2019;70(10):888–93.
6. Zerbo O, Qian Y, Ray T, et al. Health care service utilization and cost among adults with autism spectrum disorders in a u.s. integrated health care system. Autism in Adulthood 2019;1(1):27–36.
7. Zablotsky B, Pringle BA, Colpe LJ, et al. Service and treatment use among children diagnosed with autism spectrum disorders. J Dev Behav Pediatr 2015;36(2):98–105.
8. Centers for Disease Control. Autism and developmental disabilities monitoring (ADDM) network. 2021. Available at. https://www.cdc.gov/ncbddd/autism/addm.html. Accessed Retrieved December 29, 2021.
9. Dietz PM, Rose CE, McArthur D, et al. National and state estimates of adults with autism spectrum disorder. J Autism Dev Disord 2020;50(12):4258–66.
10. Hyman SL, Levy SE, Myers SM, et al. Identification, evaluation, and management of children with autism spectrum disorder. Pediatrics 2020;145(1):e20193447.
11. Reichow B, Hume K, Barton EE, et al, Reichow, B., Hume, K., Barton, E.E., et al.,. Early intensive behavioral intervention (EIBI) for young children with autism spectrum disorders (ASD). Cochrane Database Syst Rev 2018;(5):CD009260.
12. Pickles A, Le Couteur A, Leadbitter K, et al. Parent-mediated social communication therapy for young children with autism (PACT): long-term follow-up of a randomised controlled trial. Lancet 2016;388(10059):2501–9.
13. Baio J, Wiggins L, Christensen DL, et al. Prevalence of autism spectrum disorder among children aged 8 years — autism and developmental disabilities monitoring network, 11 sites, United States, 2014. MMWR Surveill Summ 2018;67(No. SS-6):1–23. https://doi.org/10.15585/mmwr.ss6706a1external icon.
14. Magaña S, Lopez K, Aguinaga A, et al. Access to diagnosis and treatment services among latino children with autism spectrum disorders. Intellect Dev Disabil 2013;51(3):141–53.
15. Mandell DS, Ittenbach RF, Levy SE, et al. Disparities in diagnoses received prior to a diagnosis of autism spectrum disorder. J Autism Dev Disord 2007;37(9):1795–802.
16. Centers for Disease Control. Data and statistics on autism spectrum disorder. 2021. Available at. https://www.cdc.gov/ncbddd/autism/data.html. Accessed December 24, 2021.
17. Bishop-Fitzpatrick L, Kind AJH. A scoping review of health disparities in autism spectrum disorder. J Autism Dev Disord 2017;47(11):3380–91.
18. Magaña S, Parish SL, Rose RA, et al. Racial and ethnic disparities in quality of health care among children with autism and other developmental disabilities. Intellect Dev Disabil 2012;50(4):287–99.
19. Constantino JN, Abbacchi AM, Saulnier C, et al. Timing of the diagnosis of autism in african american children. Pediatrics 2020;146(3). e20193629.
20. Mandell DS, Wiggins LD, Carpenter LA, et al. Racial/ethnic disparities in the identification of children with autism spectrum disorders. Am J Public Health 2009;99:493–8.
21. Elder JH, Brasher S, Alexander B. Identifying the barriers to early diagnosis and treatment in underserved individuals with autism spectrum disorders (ASD) and their families: a qualitative study. Issues Ment Health Nurs 2016;37(6):412–20.

22. Healthy People. Disparities. 2021. Available at: https://www.healthypeople.gov/2020/about/foundation-health-measures/Disparities. Accessed January 15, 2022.
23. National Institute on Minority Health and Health Disparities (2021). Available at: https://www.nimhd.nih.gov/about/overview/. Accessed December 29, 2021.
24. Manuel JI. Racial/ethnic and gender disparities in health care use and access. Health Serv Res 2018;53(3):1407–29. Epub 2017 May 8. PMID: 28480588; PMCID: PMC5980371.
25. Nichols HM, Dababnah S, Troen B, et al. Racial disparities in a sample of inpatient youth with ASD. Autism Res 2020;13(4):532–8.
26. Bilaver LA, Sobotka SA, Mandell DS. Understanding racial and ethnic disparities in autism-related service use among medicaid-enrolled children. J Autism Dev Disord 2021;51(9):3341–55.
27. Bilaver LA, Havlicek J. Racial and ethnic disparities in autism-related health and educational services. J Dev Behav Pediatr 2019;40(7):501–10.
28. Ennis-Cole D, Durodoye BA, Harris HL. The impact of culture on autism diagnosis and treatment: considerations for counselors and other professionals. Fam J 2013;21(3):279–87.
29. Broder-Fingert S, Mateo C, Zuckerman KE. Structural racism and autism. Pediatrics 2020;146(3). e2020015420.
30. Centers for Disease Control. Spotlight on closing the racial and ethnic gaps in the identification of autism spectrum disorder among 8-year-old children. 2021. Available at: https://www.cdc.gov/ncbddd/autism/addm-community-report/spotlight-on-closing-racial-gaps.html. Accessed December 26, 2021.
31. Magaña S, Parish SL, Son E. Functional severity and Latino ethnicity in specialty services for children with autism spectrum disorder: Severity and Latino children with ASD. J Intellect Disabil Res 2016;60(5):424–34.
32. Iadarola S, Pellecchia M, Stahmer A, et al. Mind the gap: an intervention to support caregivers with a new autism spectrum disorder diagnosis is feasible and acceptable. Pilot Feasibility Stud 2020;6(1):124.
33. Schott W, Tao S, Shea L. Co-occurring conditions and racial-ethnic disparities: medicaid enrolled adults on the autism spectrum. Autism Res 2022;15(1):70–85.
34. Croen LA, Zerbo O, Qian Y, et al. The health status of adults on the autism spectrum. Autism 2015;19(7):814–23.
35. Vohra R, Madhavan S, Sambamoorthi U. Emergency department use among adults with autism spectrum disorders (ASD). J Autism Dev Disord 2016;46(4):1441–54.
36. Gardner L, Campbell JM, Westdal J. Brief Report: Descriptive analysis of law enforcement officers' experiences with and knowledge of autism. J Autism Dev Disord 2019;49(3):1278–83.
37. Hinkle KA, Lerman DC. Preparing law enforcement officers to engage successfully with individuals with autism spectrum disorder: an evaluation of a performance-based approach. J Autism Dev Disord 2021. https://doi.org/10.1007/s10803-021-05192-5.
38. Rava J, Shattuck P, Rast J, et al. The prevalence and correlates of involvement in the criminal justice system among youth on the autism spectrum. J Autism Dev Disord 2017;47(2):340–6.
39. Palumba J. Why you should care about black autistic lives and CESSA 2020. Forbes. Retrieved from. https://www.forbes.com/sites/jenniferpalumbo/2020/09/01/black-autistic-lives-matter/?sh=2d36f65b427d. Accessed January 21, 2022.
40. Nicolaidis C, Kripke CC, Raymaker D. Primary care for adults on the autism spectrum. Med Clin North Am 2014;98(5):1169–91.

41. Brasher S, Middour-Oxler B, Chambers R, et al. Caring for Adults with autism spectrum disorder in the emergency department: lessons learned from pediatric emergency colleagues. J Emerg Nurs 2021;47(3):384–9.
42. Schott W, Verstreate K, Tao S, et al. Autism grows up: medicaid's role in serving adults on the spectrum. Psychiatr Serv 2021;72(5):597.
43. Farley M, Cottle KJ, Bilder D, et al. Mid-life social outcomes for a population-based sample of adults with ASD. Autism Res 2018;11(1):142–52.
44. Stahmer AC, Vejnoska S, Iadarola S, et al. Caregiver voices: Cross-cultural input on improving access to autism services. J Racial Ethnic Health Disparities 2019; 6(4):752–73. https://doi.org/10.1007/s40615-019-00575-y. Available at:.
45. Muirhead L, Brasher S, Broadnax D, et al. A framework for evaluating SDOH curriculum integration. J Prof Nurs 2022;39:1–9.
46. Hassan MM, Mokhtar HMO. Investigating autism etiology and heterogeneity by decision tree algorithm. Inform Med Unlocked 2019;16:100215.
47. Autism Association of Western Australia. Common misconceptions. 2022. Available at: https://www.autism.org.au/what-is-autism/common-misconceptions/. Accessed January 22, 2022.
48. Department of human & health services aging and disability services division. Autism myths and misconceptions. (n.d.). Available at: https://adsd.nv.gov/uploadedFiles/adsdnvgov/content/Programs/Autism/ATAP/Autism%20Myths%20and%20Misconceptions.pdf. Accessed January 20, 2022.
49. Lai MC, Lombardo MV, Ruigrok AN, et al. Quantifying and exploring camouflaging in men and women with autism. Autism 2017;21(6):690–702.